Nutrition Specialist Certification Exam Study Guide

*by Dr. Jane Pentz
and Michael McElveen*
http://aasdn.org/
info@aasdn.org

Cover Designed By The Fred Group, LLC

Nutrition Specialist Certification Exam

Study Guide

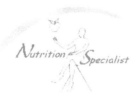

Printed in the United States of America
ISBN: 978-1-892426-23-9
Contact Information:
info@AASDN.org
http://aasdn.org/

Introduction

The American Academy of Sports Dietitians and Nutritionists (AASDN) Advisory Committee has defined the major domains of performance, the tasks associated with knowledge, skills and abilities necessary to perform the tasks required by Nutrition Specialists. The AASDN-NS Job Analysis Study defines the current knowledge, skills and abilities that must be demonstrated by AASDN Nutrition Specialist certification holders to safely and successfully practice the profession.

The latest job analysis survey was completed by Lifestyle Management Associates in June of 2005. Lifestyle Management Associates appointed an advisory committee (LMA-AC) of subject matter experts in the fitness and nutrition fields to represent Nutrition Specialists (personal trainers that incorporate nutrition education). The purpose of the LMA-AC was to construct and validate the Nutrition Specialist Examination. The committee consisted of 6 subject matter experts. These experts represented a variety of education levels and experience in the fitness and nutrition fields.

The five performance domains (statistically weighted) identified by the LMA-AC include:

Performance Domains	Weight
The Science of Nutrition	19%
Incorporating Nutrition Programs	20%
Communication/Coaching Skills	23%
Nutrition Research – Applications and Methods	21%
Professional and Legal Practices	17%

The statistically weighted performance domains were used to produce the exam content outline.

This study guide and activity workbook provides students with:
- Details concerning the Nutrition Specialist candidate policy and exam policy
- Nutrition Specialist recertification/renewal policy, scope of practice and professional code of conduct
- Study questions encompassing the material necessary to successfully complete the Nutrition Specialist Exam
- Answers to the study questions
- Study **activities/workbook** for each of the 5 performance domains designed to reinforce the skills needed for successful completion of the AASDN Nutrition Specialist exam

- Examples of Nutrition Specialist Certification exam questions

AASDN Mission Statement

The American Academy of Sports Dietitians and Nutritionists (AASDN) is a non-profit organization dedicated to providing sound, scientific, nutrition education, certifications, and resources to health and fitness professionals.

In furtherance of the AASDN mission, AASDN is the first national organization to recognize the achievements of licensed dietitians and nutritionists who possess extensive experience and education in a fitness/wellness related field. These highly qualified and experienced professionals are equipped to monitor programs implemented by other professionals. This process permits implementation of safe, effective, scientific nutrition programs by professionals that adhere to all state licensure.

Also in furtherance of this mission, AASDN has established the AASDN Nutrition Specialist Certification Program. The Nutrition Specialist certification advances professional standards through rigorous training. These highly trained Nutrition Specialists incorporate nutrition into their programs using materials developed by AASDN licensed professionals. Nutrition Specialist programs are also monitored by AASDN licensed professionals.

AASDN Administration

The AASDN Credentialing Commission (AASDN-CC) is the governing body of the AASDN Nutrition Specialist Certification Program. The AASDN-CC assesses the knowledge and skills required for the performance of tasks required by Nutrition Specialists.

The AASDN Credentialing Commission provides advisement on all matters pertaining to certification standards and policies, recertification standards and policies, approved continuing education policies and professional practice and disciplinary policies.

The AASDN-CC may adopt such rules and regulations for the conduct of its business and it shall deem advisable, and may, in the execution of such powers grant certain of its authority, responsibility and day-to-day operational duties to the AASDN Board of Certification (AASDN-BOC).

The AASDN-BOC and the AASDN-CC are dedicated to ensuring public health and safety by awarding the Nutrition Specialist credential to professionals that demonstrate competence through a system of rigorous testing and continuing education programs.

The AASDN-BOC serves independently to uphold the stringent standards of AASDN professional programs and monitor the integrity of these programs, and to implement the standards, guidelines and policy created by the AASDN Credentialing Commission regarding obtaining, and/or maintaining the AASDN Nutrition Specialist certification and completion of the AASDN Online Sports Nutrition Certificate Programs.

The AASDN-BOC Program Director is responsible for the addition of new programs, monitoring and improving current programs and overseeing the AASDN-BOC daily operations conducted by staff, advisers and consultants.

Certification Purpose Statement

AASDN-BOC provides a nutrition certification – The Nutrition Specialist Certification – for professionals. "Wellness professionals" refers to individuals that practice health in the context of a healthy balance of the mind, body, and spirit that results in an overall feeling of well-being and excludes licensed dietitians/nutritionists. "Fitness professional" refers to both health related and skilled related fitness professionals. "Athletic Trainers'" refers to individuals that meet the requirements of a state licensing board and qualifications set by the Board of Certification. Athletic Trainers' are under the direction of a physician and are recognized by the American Medical Association; and are in good standing with the Board of Certification and their state licensing board. For the purposes of this document "professionals" will refer to all unlicensed nutrition professionals.

Conflict of Interest

AASDN, AASDN-BOC and AASDN-CC maintain a strict Conflict of Interest Policy for its staff, volunteers and board members. AASDN has no legal or financial connection to accreditation organizations from which it seeks accreditation. AASDN-BOC has no financial or legal connections to NOCA or NCCA or any other accreditation organization.

Funding for AASDN programs is achieved through AASDN memberships and the AASDN Nutrition Specialist Certification. AASDN accepts no advertising, no corporate funds or government funds. AASDN extends its sincere gratitude to members and Nutrition Specialist certificants who provide support for all AASDN programs.

Nutrition Specialist Performance Domains

The latest job analysis survey was completed by Lifestyle Management Associates in June of 2005. Lifestyle Management Associates appointed an advisory committee (LMA-AC) of subject matter experts in the fitness and nutrition fields to represent Nutrition Specialists (personal trainers that incorporate nutrition education). The purpose of the LMA-AC was to construct and validate the Nutrition Specialist Examination. The committee consisted of 6 subject matter experts. These experts represented a variety of education levels and experience in the fitness and nutrition fields.

The five performance domains (statistically weighted) identified by the LMA-AC include:

Performance Domains*	Weight
The Science of Nutrition	19%
Incorporating Nutrition Programs	20%
Communication/Coaching Skills	23%
Nutrition Research – Applications and Methods	21%
Professional and Legal Practices	17%

* Performance Domains validated 2005 AASDN-NS Job Analysis Study

The statistically weighted performance domains were used to produce the exam content outline.

Table of Contents

Part 1
Certification

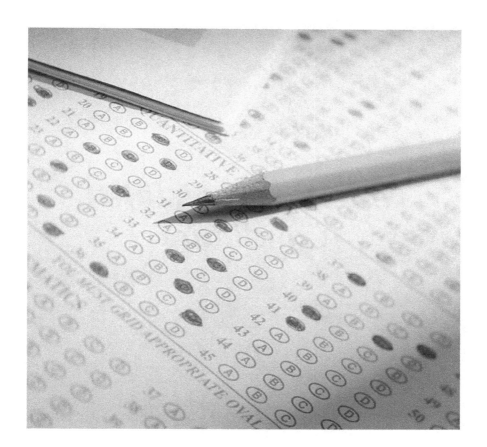

AASDN

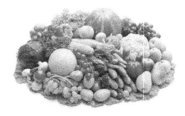

Nutrition Specialist Candidate

Nutrition Specialist Candidate

Candidates are NOT required to purchase or participate in any AASDN educational offerings and may purchase the AASDN Nutrition Specialist Exam without participation in any AASDN educational offerings. The purpose of supporting AASDN Nutrition Specialist training programs is to provide participants with options for practical application of the subject matter. Candidates enrolled in any of the AASDN training programs are not guaranteed improved performance on the exam.

Requirements Summary

A) Requirements:
   i. Candidates must be 18 years of age.
   ii. Candidates must read the Candidate Policy, Exam Policy, Rectification and Renewal Policy, Scope of Practice, and agree to the terms and conditions.
   iii. AASDN is committed to reducing obesity rates through exercise and nutrition. Candidates are not required to be certified fitness professionals or Athletic Trainers', but must work in conjunction with a certified fitness professional or a fitness facility that will be responsible for implementing an exercise component. All candidates must show proof of an exercise component by either:
   - A certificate, certification or degree in an exercise/fitness/health related field
   - Or work directly with an exercise/fitness institution
   - Or work directly with a fitness professional
   iv. Candidates must complete the online "Register for the NS Exam" form and accept the Terms and Conditions of Candidacy.
   v. Registrations must be paid in full.
B) The Nutrition Specialist Exam is an online, open book exam and is designed to test the ability of the Candidate to find and apply information and knowledge, and problem solve. Hence, Candidates are allowed access to the Nutrition for Professionals Textbook, other textbooks, study materials (open book exam) and are allowed up to 3 hours for completion of the exam.
   i. Details concerning registration for the exam can be found online at http://www.aasdn.org/ (click on "Nutrition Specialist" and then on "Exam Details").

Candidate Policy

A) Non-discrimination Policy. AASDN-BOC does not discriminate against any individual on the basis of gender, religion, ethnic background, or physical disability. Nutrition Specialist exam procedures allow for exam online completion of the examination and hence provides for accommodations for Americans with disabilities.

B) Candidate Eligibility Policy. Candidates are not required to enroll in any AASDN educational programs or purchase AASDN materials. Candidates must:

   ii. Be 18 years of age.

   iii. Must read the Candidate Policy and agree to its terms and conditions.

   iv. AASDN is committed to reducing obesity rates through exercise and nutrition. Candidates are not required to be certified fitness professionals, but must work in conjunction with a certified fitness professional or a fitness facility that will be responsible for implementing the exercise component. All candidates must show proof of an exercise component by either:
   - A certificate, certification or degree in an exercise/fitness/health related field
   - Or work directly with an exercise/fitness institution
   - Or work directly with a fitness professional

   v. Candidates must complete the registration form and accept the Terms and Conditions of Candidacy.

   vi. Registrations must be paid in full.

C) Candidate Ineligibility. A candidate may be deemed ineligible for either insufficient documentation to assess eligibility or documentation provided is incorrect, or fees do not meet eligibility requirements for the exam. The AASDN-BOC reserves the right to cancel exam scores if an individual is deemed ineligible to take the exam. If a candidate is determined to be ineligible, a refund of registration fees will NOT be provided.

D) Candidate Information Confidentiality Policy. No member of the AASDN-BOC, AASDN Credentialing Commission, AASDN-BOC employees, AASDN employees, committees or advisory committees shall divulge candidate or certified member information without express written consent from said individuals. Certified member information and confidential information consists of applications, raw certification member information, confidential numbers and email addresses. Candidates acknowledge and agree that certification status is not confidential information and that AASDN may disclose current certification status, including expiration dates, to third parties.

AASDN

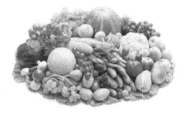

Nutrition Specialist Exam

Nutrition Specialist Exam

The Nutrition Specialist Exam is an online, open book exam and is designed to test the ability of the Candidate to find and apply information and knowledge, and problem solve. Hence, Candidates are allowed access to the Nutrition for Professionals Textbook, other textbooks, study materials (open book exam) and are allowed up to 3 hours for completion of the exam.

Exam Policy

A) Students that have completed the appropriate paperwork and paid the appropriate fees may complete the online Nutrition Specialist examination. Each exam issued will have a specific ID number.

B) Exam Completion Policy. Upon receipt by AASDN of the completed online "Register for the Exam" form, candidates will be sent an email with a Nutrition Specialist ID number, along with details on how to enter the exam site. Candidates have 6 months from the date of receipt of the Nutrition Specialist ID number to complete the exam. Candidates have the option to apply for an extension in writing. To avoid forfeiture, candidates are able to extend their exam deadline for an additional 90 days from the expiration date. Candidates that fail to apply for an extension will nullify certification candidacy. Extension requests must be approved prior to the 6 month expiration date. A $50 extension fee to extend the examination deadline must be purchased. Only one extension may be purchased. The extension period will begin from the 6 month expiration date through an additional 90 days. Extensions can be purchased online at http://www.aasdnstore.com (click on Nutrition Specialist Exam).

C) Exam Completion Details. Candidates are expected to conduct themselves in an ethical manner while completing the exam. Candidates and are not allowed to share, discuss, in any form or manner the contents of the AASDN Nutrition Specialist Certification Exam. Sharing of any information contained the AASDN Nutrition Specialist Exam is in direct violation of Federal Copyright laws governing AASDN published materials. Violations of the confidentiality agreement will result in suspension or revocation of the AASDN Nutrition Specialist Certification. To maintain security and integrity of the AASDN Nutrition Specialist Exam, examination materials are not available for review.

D) Exam Confidentiality Policy. Exam questions and content are not available for review. AASDN will not discuss exam questions with the candidate or third parties.

E) Exam Scoring Policy. Candidates must receive a score of 75 or greater to pass the exam.

F) Exam Results Reporting. Candidates receive immediate scores, a temporary certification certificate, and membership details upon completion of the exam. Printable certification certificates and membership details are mailed within 21 days of successful completion of the exam.

G) Exam Disciplinary Action. Candidates may be refused the Nutrition Specialist Certification if: he/she obtained or attempted to obtain the certification by fraud, deception or artifice; knowingly assisted in obtaining or attempting to obtain certification by fraud, deception or artifice; illegally used or falsified certification certificate, credential or any other AASDN document; knowingly obtained or received unauthorized possession and/or distribution of any official Nutrition Specialist testing materials which included copying, reproducing in any manner any part of the Nutrition Specialist exam which includes AASDN or certification logos. Candidates may be refused the Nutrition Specialist certification if the completed exam does not adhere to details specified online at http://www.aasdn.org (click on "Nutrition Specialist" and then on "Exam Details").

H) Exam Results Appeal. To maintain the security and integrity of the exam, exam materials are not available for review. Candidates may send written appeal to the AASDN-BOC. Address all appeals to the address on the AASDN website - www.aasdn.org. Requests must be made no later than 30 days following the release of the examination results. Requests received later than 30 days will not be processed. AASDN-CC will provide a response to appeals within 60 days of receipt of written appeal. Decisions by the AASDN-CC will be considered final.

I) Request to retake the exam. Candidates that do not pass the exam may reapply after a 60 day waiting period. There is a $125 fee associated with retaking the exam. Candidates that do not pass the exam a second time may not reapply for 6 months and must begin the candidacy procedure again and pay full fees.

J) Application Expiration. Upon receipt by AASDN of the completed online "Register for the Exam" form, candidates will be sent an email with a Nutrition Specialist ID number, along with details on how to enter the exam site. Candidates have 6 months from the date of receipt of the Nutrition Specialist ID number to complete the exam. Candidates have the option to apply for an extension in writing. To avoid forfeiture, candidates are able to extend their exam deadline for an additional 90 days from the expiration date. Candidates that fail to apply for an extension will nullify certification candidacy. Extension requests must be approved prior to the 6 month expiration date. A $50 extension fee to extend the examination deadline must be purchased. Only one extension may be purchased. The extension period will begin from the 6 month expiration date through an additional 90 days. Extensions can be purchased online at http://www.aasdnstore.com (click on Nutrition Specialist Exam).

K) Maintain/Update Personal Information. It is the responsibility of all candidates to notify AASDN of status and address changes before materials are shipped or attending workshops. Candidates may update their information by phone by completing the change of address form in the online member center.

L) Examination Cancellation and Refund Policy. Exam purchases and extensions are nonrefundable.

M) Workshop Cancellation/Refund/Transfer Policy. Candidates choosing the Live Workshop program must comply with the refund and continuing education policy. The purpose of a workshop is to provide participants with a live, practical application of the subject matter but is not a guarantee of improved performance on the Nutrition Specialist Exam. Space is limited so preregistration is required. A $10 late fee is added for registrations received 10 days prior to the class date. A refund is given for cancellations with 30 days notice prior to the live workshop date; however, a charge of $50 will be applied for handling/shipping charges. Additional charges will be applied for materials not returned. All returned items must be in "saleable" condition. All other cancellations will be credited toward future workshops. A $50 charge will be applied for changing/switching course dates. A 24-hour notice is required for any credit toward future workshops. No-shows who do not arrive at the workshop and who do not cancel or transfer their registrations will forfeit the registration fee. Should they wish to take the workshop at a later date they will need to register again and pay the full registration fee. Should fewer than 10 candidates register for a workshop, AASDN and Lifestyle Management Associates retain the right to cancel the workshop. Those affected will be notified no later than 7 days before the workshop date and offered the opportunity to transfer to a different site at no additional cost; obtain a refund; or switch to the home study course. Neither Lifestyle Management Associates nor AASDN is responsible for expenses incurred by a candidate due to a canceled workshop.

N) AASDN is committed to attaining and maintaining high standards as a continuing education provider. Therefore, students must attend the entire workshop to receive continuing education.

Fee Structures/Deadlines

Fee Structure	FEE
Extension Fee	$50.00
Retake Fee	$125.00
Workshop Rescheduling Fee	$50.00
Practice Exam Fee	$50.00
Prices subject to change without notice	

NS Annual Renewal Fee	FEE
Basic Fee (Due by December 31st)	$35.00
Late Fee (Jan 1st through Jan 31st)	$50.00
Late Fee (Feb 1st through Dec. 31st)	$75.00
Termination (After one Year Grace Period)	Must Recertify
Prices subject to change without notice	

Deadlines

Form	Deadline Date
Nutrition Specialist exam completion	6 months from date of receipt
Notification of exam results	Immediately upon completion of exam
Receipt of NS certificate	30 days upon completion of exam
Examination extension	90 day from exam expiration date
Retaking the exam	Waiting period of 60 days from notification
Retaking the exam (third time)	Waiting period of 6 months from notification
Breach of examination security	One year from notification of breach of security
Examination disciplinary action	One year from notification of disciplinary action

Exam Form Development

The AASDN-NS Job Analysis Study defines the current knowledge, skills and abilities that must be demonstrated by AASDN Nutrition Specialist certification holders to safely and successfully practice the profession.

The last job analysis survey was completed by Lifestyle Management Associates in June of 2005. Lifestyle Management Associates appointed an advisory committee (LMA-AC) of subject matter experts in the fitness and nutrition fields to represent Nutrition Specialists (personal trainers that incorporate nutrition education). The purpose of the LMA-AC was to construct and validate the Nutrition Specialist Examination. The committee consisted of 6 subject matter experts. These experts represented a variety of education levels and experience in the fitness and nutrition fields.

The LMA-AC subject matter experts constructed the exam items. The Nutrition Specialist Exam was built by constructing items from the performance domains and according to the content outline validated by the LMA Job Analysis Study. Items were assigned to the examination form by ensuring that the items on the form matched the exam specifications by domain. All items were selected to match the statistical requirements established.

Once items were placed correctly in the form, the form was delivered to RMP (Data Analysis Manager) through a secure, password protected database. Each item underwent a strict review process to confirm correctness, readability, relevance and direct association with the content outline. The examination form was pre-tested by 10 Certificants. All items were again analyzed by the AASDN-AC. Items performing poorly were reviewed and either modified retired or left unchanged. The final form consisted of 70 scored items and 5 non-scored items (test). Items consisted of short essay, fill-in, multiple choice and true/false questions. Therefore, scoring judgments were objectively and consistently applied.

Cut Score

LMA-AC, again with the help of RMP, established a "Cut Score" for the AASDN Nutrition Specialist Certification Exam using the Angoff procedure. The LMA-AC answered all test questions. Committee members were then given the answers and reviewed their answers for each exam question. The committee then discussed the acceptable minimum level of competency necessary for a candidate to pass the exam, and reviewed the minimum knowledge, skills, and abilities (SKA's) and eligibility qualifications of the candidate who could earn the credential. Each committee member then reviewed each test question and estimated the percentage of such individuals who would answer the question correctly. A mean for each question was then calculated. The sum of all means was divided by the total number of questions. The standard deviation was 2.769 and the standard error of the cut score was 1.1. The results indicated that the observed cut score was 76. Based on these results, the cut score of 75 was implemented.

The effect of following the Angoff procedure takes into account the difficulty of each test question and provides a standard that is not dependent on a particular group of test takers, and establishes a fully defensible cut score determination.

Exam Content

The AASDN-NS Job Analysis Study defines the current knowledge, skills and abilities that must be demonstrated by AASDN Nutrition Specialist certification holders to safely and successfully practice the profession.

The last job analysis survey was completed by Lifestyle Management Associates in June of 2005. Lifestyle Management Associates appointed an advisory committee (LMA-AC) of subject matter experts in the fitness and nutrition fields to represent Nutrition Specialists (personal trainers that incorporate nutrition education). The purpose of the LMA-AC was to construct and validate the Nutrition Specialist Examination. The committee consisted of 6 subject matter experts. These experts represented a variety of education levels and experience in the fitness and nutrition fields.

The five performance domains (statistically weighted) identified by the LMA-AC include:

Performance Domains*	Weight
The Science of Nutrition	19%
Incorporating Nutrition Programs	20%
Communication/Coaching Skills	23%
Nutrition Research – Applications and Methods	21%
Professional and Legal Practices	17%

* Performance Domains validated 2005 AASDN-NS Job Analysis Study

The statistically weighted performance domains were used to produce the exam content outline.

Domain 1 – The Science of Nutrition

This domain ensures that the Nutrition Specialist has the knowledge and skill to adequately answer questions pertaining to: the biology of cells; nutrition basics including the Recommended Dietary Allowances, Dietary Reference Intakes, and the national food guidance system; metabolism, digestion, absorption, and transport of the energy nutrients; energy production and utilization; nutrition and disease; vitamins and minerals; and complementary and alternative medicine.

Domain 2 – Incorporating Nutrition Programs

This domain ensures that the Nutrition Specialist has the necessary skills to implement a nutrition program in conjunction with a fitness/wellness program. This domain focuses on skills necessary to work with clients including the steps involved in implementation of an individual nutrition program; a group program; a child and teen program; a program for seniors, athletes, and vegetarians. The Nutrition Specialist must also possess the skills necessary to educate clients on sabotaging factors in maintaining health. Such factors include: why diets lead to muscle loss; inconsistencies and often ambiguous labeling regulations that lead to poor food choices; eating out that also leads to poor eating choices; and other sabotaging effects such as friendly saboteurs and distortion of portion sizes, etc.

Domain 3 – Communication/Coaching Skills

Coaching and counseling are allied fields that share the goal of helping clients achieve lives of greater health and fulfillment. Both counselors and coaches help clients set measurable, attainable goals. Both teach the skills necessary for achieving the goals and both provide support and encouragement while clients work toward their goals. A major difference is the client population. Coaches work with clients who are reasonably healthy and well-functioning and wish to augment their well-being through achieving certain personal or professional goals. Goals may be specific to wellness or performance or may be more broadly aimed at achieving greater life satisfaction through, for example, changes in career or lifestyle. Coaching is focused on the present and its influence on the future. The work is also typically brief and designed to accomplish the client's goals relatively quickly. "Improvement" and "enhancement" are hallmarks of coaching. Hence, all Nutrition Specialists must understand the differences between coaching and counseling and must acquire a working knowledge of coaching skills in order to help clients set measurable, attainable goals and teach the skills necessary for achieving those goals.

Domain 4 – Nutrition Research – Applications and Methods

The revolution in genetics, patent protections for bio-engineered molecules, laws strengthening intellectual property rights, and licensing and patenting of results from federally-sponsored research have created new incentives for scientists, clinicians, and academic institutions to join forces with for-profit industry in an unprecedented array of entrepreneurial activities. While many professionals are involved in research, many more read the results of research and apply it to the real world. Therefore, it is vitally important for the Nutrition Specialist to be able to critically analyze research to determine if the methods and results are valid, and to be able to disseminate sound, scientific nutrition information to the public.

Domain 5 – Professional and Legal Practices

The AASDN Nutrition Specialist Certification is the only non-regulatory nutrition certification program that includes all materials used by certificants including administrative documents; scripted programs; and unlimited sports dietitian support. The American Academy of Sports Dietitians and Nutritionists (AASDN) has undertaken the task of developing a more specific nutrition scope of practice for AASDN Nutrition Specialists (NS). This scope of practice is applicable to all non-licensed professionals that partner with qualified, licensed professionals but is specific to AASDN certified professionals. The goal of this domain is to provide AASDN certificants with clear, concise, and professional standards for inclusion of nutrition education. These guidelines are aimed at clarifying issues and adherence to all state nutrition licensure laws. Hence, this domain ensures that the AASDN Nutrition Specialist Certification program standards provide safe, effective and legal programs to the public; and that the Nutrition Specialist will continue to improve in competence in the profession through a professional code of conduct, maintain competence through continuing education, and adhere to a defined scope of practice.

AASDN

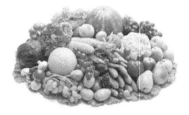

Nutrition Specialist Recertification / Renewal Policy

Recertification/Renewal Policy

Due to the rapid advances in nutrition research and addition of nutritional products AASDN Credentialing Commission has determined that recertification of the Nutrition Specialist Certification every two years is warranted. The purpose of recertification is to ensure that qualified professionals maintain and enhance levels of proficiency in their related fields through continuing education requirements. Continuing education programs promote continuing development of expertise and skills.

Rectification Policy

To support AASDN's commitment to dissemination of sound, scientific information to the public, maintaining the Nutrition Specialist certification includes the following:

- AASDN requires a total of 15 contact hours every two years. Content must fall within the Domains listed in the table below. AASDN also accepts documentation of work in the field of nutrition such as nutrition classes, lectures, etc. Certificants must complete the online Continuing Education Course Petition form for approval of work completed in the field of nutrition. The five performance domains (statistically weighted) identified by the LMA-AC include:

Performance Domains*	Weight
The Science of Nutrition	19%
Incorporating Nutrition Programs	20%
Communication/Coaching Skills	23%
Nutrition Research – Applications and Methods	21%
Professional and Legal Practices	17%

- Nutrition Specialists are not required to recertify until the next reporting period following certification. For example, a certificant that successfully completed the Nutrition Specialist exam in 2014 is not required to recertify until the 2017 reporting period.

Reporting Period	
2013	January 1st 2012 through December 31st 2013
2015	January 1st 2014 through December 31st 2015
2017	January 1st 2016 through December 31st 2017
2019	January 1st 2018 through December 31st 2019

- CECs are based on contact hours. Contact hours are defined as the number of actual clock hours spent in direct participation in a structured educational format as a learner. One (1) CEC is equivalent to one (1) contact hour. CECs will be awarded only for activities that are completed within the reporting period. CECs in excess of the amount required cannot be carried over for credit in subsequent reporting periods. CECs cannot be earned prior to certification.
- Changes in mailing address must be provided to the AASDN-BOC. Failure to keep the mailing address current can result in suspension or revocation of certification. Information can be updated by completing the Contact Form in the member center at www.aasdn.org.
- All AASDN Certificants are held to higher standards since all Certificants are members of the health community. Therefore, AASDN-BOC has instituted a random audit whereby 10% of all Nutrition Specialists will be asked to provide documentation of contact hours. No fees are associated with this process. Certificants that are chosen will be notified via USPS and must show proof of contact hours within 60 days of notification.
- All Nutrition Specialist NOT chosen by the random audit will NOT be required to submit documentation of contact hours but are required to complete the "AASDN-BOC recertification Documentation Form" and maintain a copy for their records.

Renewal Policy

All Nutrition Specialists are required to renew their Nutrition Specialist Certification annually and have the option to switch between the 2 following membership options:

- Basic Membership. Benefits include entry into the NS member center which includes all documents needed to incorporate a nutrition program. Documents include: administrative documents, caloric needs assessment sheet; legal waiver, physician release form, responsibility agreement; ten session outline; individual scripted program, group scripted program, youth program, athletes and vegetarian program; menu plans, goal setting sheet and more.
    - Benefits also include AASDN product discounts and listing on the AASDN NS state page.
    - Benefits also include unlimited access to a sports dietitian.
    - The Basic Membership annual fee is $35 (price subject to change without notice).
- Nutrition Manager Membership. All Nutrition Specialists have the option to upgrade to the Nutrition Manager Membership at any time. This option includes

all the benefits of the basic membership and also includes the ability to provide more specialized services. AASDN professionals not only answers all questions, but also provide monitoring of client programs. For more details on this membership see Nutrition Manager at www.aasdn.org. The membership fee for Nutrition Manager is $299 annually (price subject to change without notice).

AASDN

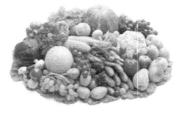

Nutrition Specialist Scope of Practice

Nutrition Specialist Scope of Practice

This scope of practice is applicable to all non-licensed professionals that partner with qualified, licensed professionals but is specific to AASDN certified professionals. The goal of this document is to provide AASDN certificants with clear, concise, and professional standards for inclusion of nutrition education. These guidelines are aimed at clarifying issues and adherence to all state nutrition licensure laws.

STANDARD 1: Declarations and Definitions

"AASDN" refers to the American Academy of Sports Dietitians & Nutritionists. "Board" refers to the AASDN Credentialing Commission Board members. "Wellness professionals" refers to individuals that practice health in the context of a healthy balance of the mind, body, and spirit that results in an overall feeling of well-being (16) and excludes licensed dietitians/nutritionists. "Fitness professional" refers to both health related and skilled related fitness professionals. "Athletic Trainers'" refers to individuals that meet the requirements of a state licensing board and qualifications set by the Board of Certification. Athletic Trainers' are under the direction of a physician and are recognized by the American Medical Association; and are in good standing with the Board of Certification and their state licensing board (17). "Nutrition Specialist" refers to a person who has successfully completed the AASDN Nutrition Specialist program and is a member in good standing with the AASDN Credentialing Commission. A "medical condition" is a broad term that includes all diseases and disorders (15). The "profession" refers to the profession of nutrition in conjunction with wellness programming. "Licensed professional" refers to a licensed dietitian/nutritionist.

STANDARD 2: Code of Ethics

Individuals that engage in the practice of nutrition in conjunction with fitness/wellness programming shall adhere to the AASDN Code of Ethics. The Code provides guidance for decision-making concerning ethical matters and serves as a means for self-evaluation and reflection regarding the ethical practice of nutrition in conjunction with fitness/wellness programming.

1. Accurately communicate and provide educational services equitably to all individuals regardless of social or economic status, age, gender, race, ethnicity, national origin, religion, disability, diverse values, attitudes, or opinions.
2. Be accountable for individual non-medical judgments and decisions about health and fitness, nutrition, preventive, rehabilitative, education, and/or research

services.

3. Maintain high quality professional competence through continued study of the latest research in nutrition and health and fitness as provided through respected, reliable sources.

4. Be expected to conduct educational activities in accordance with recognized legal, scientific, ethical, and professional standards.

5. Respect and protect the privacy, rights, and dignity of all individuals by not disclosing health and fitness, nutrition, and or research information unless required by law or when confidentiality jeopardizes the health and safety of others.

6. Call attention to unprofessional services that result from incompetent, unethical, or illegal professional behavior.

7. Contribute to the ongoing development and integrity of the profession by being responsive to, mutually supportive of, and accurately communicating academic and other qualifications to colleagues and associates in the field.

8. Participate in the profession's efforts to establish high quality services by avoiding conflicts of interest and endorsements of products and supplements.

9. Participate in and encourage critical discourse to reflect the collective knowledge and be proactive within the exercise and nutrition profession to protect the public from misinformation, incompetence, and unethical acts.

10. Provide interventions grounded in a theoretical framework supported by research that enables a healthy lifestyle.

STANDARD 3: Practice of Nutrition

The practice of nutrition education in conjunction with fitness/wellness programming by AASDN Nutrition Specialists shall include a variety of educational activities/documents but only when created by, reviewed by, and/or in consultation with an AASDN licensed dietitian/nutritionist. No program/document change can be initiated without prior approval by an AASDN licensed dietitian/nutritionist. No program/document can be modified or altered in any way without approval by an AASDN licensed dietitian/nutritionist. The AASDN Nutrition Specialist, in conjunction with the AASDN licensed professional, may provide clients with educational information through lectures, articles, and classes. The AASDN Nutrition Specialist, in conjunction with the AASDN licensed professional, may utilize AASDN approved documents with the apparently healthy, exercising population. Nothing in this standard authorizes the AASDN Nutrition Specialist to "diagnose" disease or make nutritional recommendations for individuals requiring special dietary needs. Nothing in this standard authorizes the AASDN Nutrition Specialist to provide such services without direct approval and in consultation with an AASDN licensed dietitian/nutritionist. The

AASDN Nutrition Specialist **cannot** provide nutrition services to individuals with medical conditions without direct oversight and in consultation with an AASDN licensed dietitian/nutritionist.

STANDARD 4: Educational Requirements

The practice of nutrition in conjunction with the AASDN Nutrition Specialist shall include a variety of educational requirements prior to practice which includes successful completion of the AASDN Nutrition Specialist Certification; and all certificants must be members in good standing with the AASDN Credentialing Commission. AASDN requires recertification of the Nutrition Specialist certification every two years. All Nutrition Specialists are required to obtain 15 contact hours every two years. All AASDN Certificants are held to higher standards since all Certificants are members of the health community. Therefore, AASDN-BOC has instituted a random audit whereby 10% of all Nutrition Specialists will be asked to provide documentation of contact hours. No fees are associated with this process. Certificants that are chosen will be notified via USPS and must show proof of contact hours within 60 days of notification.

STANDARD 5: Endorsement/Sales of Nutritional Products

AASDN does not endorse any particular supplements or brand of supplements. It is beyond the scope of practice for Nutrition Specialists to recommend or suggest the use of any nutrition supplementation (vitamin, mineral, herbal, ergogenic, or weight loss). Any such recommendations must come directly from the client's physician or a licensed dietitian. The Nutrition Specialist shall refrain from endorsement of, or sales of, supplements and products containing supplement on the label. Such endorsement or sales constitutes a conflict of interest and is beyond the scope of practice of a non-licensed professional.

STANDARD 6: Professional Responsibility/Competence

The AASDN Nutrition Specialist that has attained the AASDN Nutrition Specialist Certification who is in good legal and professional standing with all academic and certificate programs may implement programs that have been created by an AASDN licensed dietitian/nutritionist when working with the apparently, healthy exercising population. It is the responsibility of the AASDN Nutrition Specialist to be aware of specific statues in his/her state as well as understanding his/her professional standard of care and limitations in working with at risk populations or individuals with medical conditions. The AASDN Nutrition Specialist shall practice only within the boundaries of their competence as defined by their academic training, hands-on experience, professional certification, and in conjunction with a licensed dietitian/nutritionist. When indicated, the **AASDN** Nutrition Specialist professional shall monitor his/her effectiveness and take steps including, but not limited to, continuing education to maintain a reasonable level of awareness of current scientific and professional information.

Professional Code of Conduct

The AASDN Professional Code of Conduct is designed to maintain the highest level of professional and ethical conduct. AASDN-BOC expects each Nutrition Specialist to uphold the AASDN-BOC Professional Code of Conduct and Scope of Practice in its entirety. Failure to comply with the Professional Code of Conduct and Scope of Practice may result in disciplinary action including, but not limited to, suspension or termination of certification. All Certificants are obligated to report any unethical behavior or violation of the Professional Code of Conduct and Scope of Practice by other Certificants.

Each certified Nutrition Specialist must provide professional service and demonstrate safe and effective client care in their practice. Each member shall:

- Abide by the AAASD-BOC Professional Code of Conduct, including but not limited to, refraining from illegal use of terms such as dietitian and nutritionist.
- Abide by the AASDN-BOC Scope of Practice. Including, but not limited to, using materials developed by qualified professionals and refraining from recommending or selling supplements which is beyond the scope of practice for all Nutrition Specialists.
- Treat each colleague and/or client with the utmost and dignity and dignity and not make false or derogatory assumptions concerning their practice.
- Refer clients to the appropriate medical practitioner when the Nutrition Specialist becomes aware of any change in the client's health status or medication; become aware of an undiagnosed illness, injury, or risk factor; become aware of any unusual client eating behaviors. Also refer the client to appropriate health care provider when supplemental advice is requested.
- Remain in good standing and maintain current certification status by acquiring all necessary continuing education requirements.

Confidentiality

Each certified Nutrition Specialist shall respect the confidentiality of all client information. In his/her professional role, the Nutrition Specialist shall: protect the client's confidentiality in conversations, advertisement and any other arena unless otherwise agreed upon by the client in writing or due medical and/or legal necessity; protect the interests of clients who are minors by law or unable to give voluntary consent by securing the legal permission of the appropriate third party or legal guardian; store and dispose of client records in a secure manner.

Integrity

Each Nutrition Specialist must practice with honesty, integrity and lawfulness. The Nutrition Specialist shall: Maintain adequate and truthful progress notes for each client; accurately and truthfully inform the public of services rendered; honestly and truthfully represent all professional qualifications and affiliations; advertise in a manner that is honest, dignified and representative of services that can be delivered without the use of provocative and/or sexual language and or pictures.

Revocation of Certification

AASDN-BOC may revoke or otherwise take action with regard to the application or certification of an individual in the case of:

a)   Ineligibility for certification.

b)   Irregularity in connection with any certification application or examination.

c)   Unauthorized possession, use, access or distribution of certification examinations, score reports, answer sheets, certificates, Certificant or applicant files, documents or other materials. Material misrepresentation or fraud in any statement to AASDN or in any statement to the public in connection with professional practice, including, but not limited to, statements made to assist the applicant, Certificant, or another to apply for, obtain or retain certification.

d)   Negligence or malpractice in professional work, which includes, but is not limited to, the release of confidential medical information of clients or others with whom the Certificant or applicant has a professional relationship.

e)   The conviction of, plea of guilty or plea of no contest to a felony or misdemeanor, which is directly related to public health, athletic care or education. This includes but is not limited to rape, sexual abuse of a child, adult, or athlete, actual or threatened use of a weapon of violence; the prohibited sale or distribution of controlled substance, or its possession with the intent to distribute.

f)   Not adhering to the eligibility requirements for certification candidacy, including breach of exam security; or not adhering to the continuing education requirements.

g)   Not adhering to the Professional Code of Conduct and Scope of Practice.

h)   Not cooperating with AASDN and/or AASDN Credentialing Commission investigations into alleged illegal or unethical activities. This would include but is not limited to, not cooperating with appropriate committees by withholding information, not responding to requests for information in a timely manner, or providing misleading information to an AASDN committee or individual member.

i)   Engaging in conduct that includes, but is not limited to, unauthorized use of the

AASDN name to endorse any products or services without proper authority or exploitation of a client for financial gain.

Disciplinary Hearing and Appeals Panels

a) AASDN-BOC Manager shall appoint three persons who are AASDN-BOC certified professionals to a Hearing Panel, and/or an Appeals Panel, to consider alleged violations of any Application or Certification standard set forth in Section I C (1)-(7) after review and decision by the Professional Practice and Discipline Committee. These panels may be established as standing panels. The Hearing and Appeals panels shall be composed of three full voting members and up to four non-voting (substitute) members.

b) A quorum of either the Committee or a panel consists of three full voting members, and Committee and Panel action shall be determined by a majority vote. Committee and Panel members may not serve in any situation where their impartiality or the presence of actual or apparent conflict of interest might reasonably be questioned.

c) When a vacancy of a full-voting member occurs in any of the panels as a result of resignation, unavailability, or disqualification, the AASDN-BOC Manager shall designate a full voting Nutrition Specialist certified professional from the list of substitute members.

Complaint/Review Process

Whenever the AASDN-BOC Manager receives allegations that raise an issue the AASDN-BOC Manager shall transmit such allegations to the Chair of the AASDN Credentialing Commission which shall act as the Hearing Panel. The Hearing Panel shall review the complaint and contact the accuser by telephone or via postal mail to set up a time and date to review the allegation. All phone conversations will be recorded and all parties will be notified of the recording procedures. Accusers will be questioned about the facts regarding the alleged incident(s) and information relevant to the case such as times, date and location of the offense shall be reviewed with the accuser for clarity. After all those involved in the accusation are questioned, the Hearing Panel will determine if good cause exists to move further into the investigation. If the Hearing Panel determines that no good cause exists to question eligibility or compliance with the Professional Code of Conduct and Scope of Practice, no further action shall be taken. However, if the Hearing Panel determines by majority vote that good cause does exist, it shall direct the transmittal to the applicant or Certificant by certified mail or tracked courier, return receipt requested, of a letter containing a statement of the factual allegations constituting the alleged violation and the disciplinary standard allegedly violated. The letter shall also include the following recitation of rights and procedures: The applicant or Certificant shall have fifteen (15) days in which to respond to the allegations, provide comments regarding appropriate sanctions, and request a formal hearing if he or she disputes the allegations; sanctions may be imposed if the allegations are determined to be true by the Hearing Panel, or if the applicant or Certificant fails to submit a timely response; the applicant or Certificant will be deemed to consent to the imposition of sanctions by the Hearing Panel if he or she does not dispute the truthfulness of the allegations; the applicant or Certificant must appear in person if he/she requests a hearing.

Appeals

If the applicant or Certificant disputes the allegations and requests a hearing, the Chair shall: forward the allegations and response of the applicant or Certificant to the hearing panel; schedule a hearing before the Hearing Panel after the request is received; send by certified mail or tracked courier, return receipt requested, a Notice of Hearing to the applicant or Certificant. The Notice of Hearing shall include a statement of the time and place of the hearing as selected by the AASDN-BOC Manager after consultation with the Chair of the Hearing Panel. The Hearing Panel shall maintain an audio taped or written transcript of the proceedings. AASDN-BOC and the applicant or Certificant may make opening statements, present documents and testimony, examine and cross examine witnesses under oath, make closing statements and present written briefs as scheduled by the Hearing Panel.

The Hearing Panel shall determine all matters relating to the hearing. The hearing and related matters shall be determined on the record by majority vote. Formal rules of evidence shall not apply. Relevant evidence may be admitted. Disputed questions shall be determined by majority vote of the Panel. The decision of the Hearing Panel shall be rendered in writing. A decision by the Hearing Panel shall contain factual findings, conclusions of law and any sanctions applied. It shall be transmitted to the applicant or Certificant by certified mail or tracked courier, return receipt requested.

Sanctions

Sanctions for violation of any AASDN-BOC Standard may include one or more of the following: Denial or suspension of eligibility; revocation; non-renewal; censure; reprimand; suspension; training or other corrective action.

Part 2
Questions

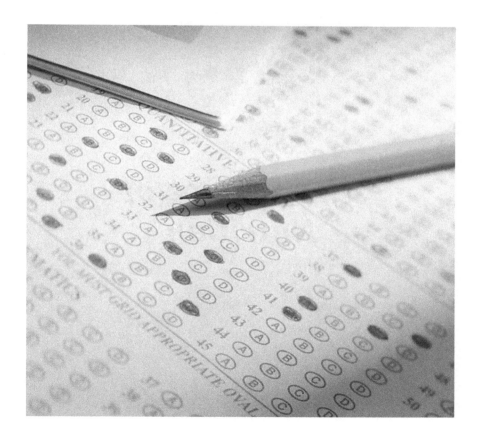

Questions

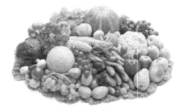

The Science of
Nutrition

Performance Domain 1- Questions
The Science of Nutrition

This domain ensures that the Nutrition Specialist has the knowledge and skill to adequately answer questions pertaining to: the biology of cells; nutrition basics including the Recommended Dietary Allowances, Dietary Reference Intakes, and the national food guidance system; metabolism, digestion, absorption and transport of the energy nutrients; energy production and utilization; nutrition and disease; vitamins and minerals; and complementary and alternative medicine.

A. Biology of Cells

Step 1 – Read pages 2 through 4 in the Nutrition for Professionals Textbook.

Step 2 – Answer the following questions:
1. How can cells be differentiated?
2. What are the differences between a prokaryotic and a eukaryotic cell?
3. List several differences between plant and animal cells.
4. List tissues found in the human body and describe each type.
5. List several differences between muscle cells, fat cells, red blood cells, and nerve cells.

B. Nutrition Basics

Step 1 – Read pages 4 through 26 in the Nutrition for Professionals Textbook.

Step 2 – Answer the following questions:
1. Define digestion and list the organs involved in the digestive system.
2. What is the role of the mucosa of the mouth, stomach and small intestines?
3. What is peristalsis? Explain the role of peristalsis in digestion of food.
4. Where does absorption of most food occur and describe the process.
5. Define digestive juices, and explain their roles.
6. Name the 3 segments of the small intestines and explain specialization of absorption of nutrients.
7. Describe the vascular and lymphatic systems and their roles in the absorption of nutrients.
8. Define calories and list the number of calories obtained from each of the energy nutrients.

9. Define anabolism and catabolism, and list the products made from the catabolism of carbohydrates, lipids, and proteins.
10. What are micronutrients?
11. Define vitamins.
12. Define minerals.
13. Define homeostasis and provide several examples.
14. Describe hormonal control of metabolism.
15. Describe the role of cellular concentration in the control of metabolism.
16. Describe the role of cellular compartmentalization in the control of metabolism.
17. Define the Dietary Reference Intake and Daily Values.
18. Define the Dietary Guidelines and provide details concerning the latest published guidelines.
19. What is the food guidance system?
20. How does the Harvard Healthy Eating Plate differ from the MyPlate icon?

C. Carbohydrates

Step 1 – Read pages 33 through 56 in the Nutrition for Professionals Textbook.

Step 2 – Answer the following questions:
1. Describe the process of carbohydrate digestion.
2. Describe the process of absorption of simple sugars.
3. What are the five fates of glucose once absorbed into the bloodstream?
4. Define glycogen and its role in energy storage as it pertains to muscle and liver.
5. Explain the process of glucose homeostasis including the hormones involved.
6. Describe the difference between insulin and noninsulin dependent cells.
7. What does the term "glucose time curve" refer to?
8. Explain the process of gluconeogenesis and its role in glucose homeostasis.
9. What is ketosis? What are ketones and how are they formed?
10. Describe the difference between absorption rate of simple sugars versus complex carbohydrates in the presence of other nutrients.
11. What is the glycemic response?
12. What is the glycemic index?
13. How does glycemic load differ from glycemic index?
14. What is insulin resistance? What are the conditions and signs associated with insulin resistance?
15. What is the treatment for insulin resistance?
16. What is fiber? What is the recommended intake, and what are the benefits of fiber in the diet?

17. Define alcohol and list possible negative and positive benefits of drinking alcoholic beverages.
18. List the categories of sweeteners and provides examples of each.

D. Lipids

Step 1 – Read pages 67 through 87 in the Nutrition for Professionals Textbook.

Step 2 – Answer the following questions:
1. Define lipids, fats, and oils.
2. List the differences between triglycerides and phospholipids, and explain the roles of each in the human body.
3. Define saturated, monounsaturated and polyunsaturated fatty acids and the differences between each.
4. What are trans fatty acids, and how are they produced? How do they differ from saturated fatty acids?
5. List the essential fatty acids and the recommended intakes for each.
6. What are eicosanoids, and what is their role in homeostasis?
7. What are prostaglandins, and explain their role in platelet aggregations?
8. What are some of the health effects of essential fatty acids in the diet?
9. Explain the problem of mercury and PCBs in fish and how to avoid these chemicals.
10. Define steroids and explain the role of cholesterol in the human body.
11. Describe the process of digestion of fats into their constituent components.
12. Describe the absorption of the constituent components of fats.
13. Describe the process of transport of fat throughout the body (packaging systems) including the exogenous and endogenous pathways.

E. Proteins

Step 1 – Read pages 93 through 106 in the Nutrition for Professionals Textbook.

Step 2 – Answer the following questions:
1. What are proteins? Explain the different types of proteins and their roles in the human body.
2. What are amino acids? Explain their roles in the human body.
3. Define and list the nonessential amino acids
4. Define and list the essential/indispensable amino acids.
5. Describe the glutamine/alanine cycle and its role as an interorgan nitrogen

carrier.

6. Define nitrogen and its role in the body.
7. Explain why nitrogen is critical to life. Describe why it is toxic and explain how the body disposes of excess nitrogen.
8. What are glucogenic and ketogenic amino acids? What are their roles in the human body?
9. Describe the digestion of proteins.
10. Explain the role of dietary protein in synthesis of body proteins.
11. Explain the absorption of amino acids.
12. Explain amino acid transport systems and the role of the blood-brain barrier in control of the central nervous system environment.
13. List the different methods of measuring protein quality and explain which method is being used today.

F. Energy

Step 1 – Read pages 115 through 141 in the Nutrition for Professionals Textbook.

Step 2 – Answer the following questions:
1. Explain the steps involved in energy productions (ATP, ATP-PC, glycolysis, TCA cycle, electron transport chain).
2. Describe each of the factors involved in energy utilization (diet, rest, exercise intensity, exercise duration, fitness level, muscle mass, catabolic factors)
3. List the percentages/grams of recommended energy nutrient intake as defined by the DRI, AND, ACSM, and the IOC.
4. List the DRI for fluids.
5. Discuss the importance of nutrient timing on athletic performance and muscle hypertrophy. List the recommendations by the AND, the ACSM, and the IOC.
6. Discuss the position stand of the AND, the ACSM, and the IOC with respect to micronutrient supplementation for athletes.
7. What are the three components for determining total energy nutrient needs?
8. Explain how the estimated energy requirements (EER) are determined for both males and females.
9. Explain how caloric needs for children are determined.
10. Explain the EER body fat adjustment.

G. Nutrition and Disease

Step 1 – Read pages 149 through 181 in the Nutrition for Professionals Textbook.

Step 2 – Answer the following questions:
1. Define diabetes and describe the stages involved in development of the disease.
2. What are the differences between the 3 main types of diabetes (Type 1 diabetes, Type 2 diabetes and gestational diabetes)?
3. How is diabetes diagnosed?
4. What are the steps in reducing diabetes risk?
5. What are some of the effects of physical activity on blood glucose levels?
6. Define cardiovascular disease?
7. What are some of the risk factors for developing heart disease?
8. What are some of the lifestyle modifications involved in reducing cardiovascular disease risk?
9. Define atherosclerosis and its role in heart disease.
10. List the levels of cholesterol, HDL and LDL associated with increased risk for cardiovascular disease.
11. What are some of the problems associated with cholesterol lowering medications?
12. What are some of the other ways to reduce cholesterol levels in addition to medications?
13. Discuss other factors involved in determining cardiovascular disease risk (L-carnitine, homocysteine, high sensitivity C-reactive protein, coronary calcium scan).
14. What is the role of physical activity in reducing cardiovascular disease risk?
15. Define hypertension and explain the method for determining disease risk.
16. What is the dash diet? What is the Mediterranean diet? What are the differences between these two diets?
17. What is the role of physical activity in reducing hypertension risk?
18. Define stroke.
19. List the factors involved in developing a stroke that can and cannot be modified.
20. What are the warning signs of stroke?
21. What is the role of physical activity in reducing the risk of stroke?
22. Which cancers may be affected by lifestyle, diet and exercise?
23. What is celiac disease, and how can it be cured?
24. What is the difference between inflammatory bowel disease and irritable bowel syndrome?
25. List the two types of inflammatory bowel disease and the differences between the two.

26. What is GERD? What are some of the factors involved in reducing the symptoms associated with GERD?
27. Define chronic kidney disease and explain how it is diagnosed.
28. List the 4 stages of kidney disease and describe each.
29. What are the dietary changes required to compensate for the reduced excretion of certain nutrients in kidney disease?

H. *Vitamins and Minerals*

Step 1 – Read pages 197 through 253 in the Nutrition for Professionals Textbook.

Step 2 – Answer the following questions:
1. List the water soluble vitamins and describe their roles in metabolism. Also include foods, recommended intakes, deficiency and toxicity symptoms.
2. List the fat soluble vitamins and describe their roles in metabolism. Also include foods, recommended intakes, deficiency and toxicity symptoms.
3. Discuss the importance of water and include recommended intake, deficiency and toxicity symptoms.
4. List the major minerals and describe their roles in metabolism. Also include foods, recommended intakes, deficiency and toxicity symptoms.
5. List the trace minerals and describe their roles in metabolism. Also include foods, recommended intakes, deficiency and toxicity symptoms.

I. *Complementary and Alternative Medicine*

Step 1 – Read pages 261 through 293 in the Nutrition for Professionals Textbook.

Step 2 – Answer the following questions:
1. Define complementary and alternative medicine.
2. What is NCCAM? Explain its role as it relates to complementary and alternative medicine.
3. What are the NCCAM classifications for complementary health approaches?
4. Define dietary supplements.
5. Define mind-body practices.
6. What caused a major increase in the use of dietary supplements? Describe the law that was passed at this time.
7. How did the supplement industry change as a result of the passage of this law?
8. What is the ODS? When and why was is created?
9. Explain how dietary supplements are now regulated.

10. List and explain the types of claims that can be made on dietary supplement labels.
11. What does standardization refer to? Explain the laws regarding standardization.
12. List the 4 categories of supplements and define each category.
13. List 8 categories of ergogenic aids and explain the pros and cons of each.
14. List 6 categories of weight loss supplements/approaches evaluated by NCCAM and describe the pros and cons of each.
15. List and discuss three supplement verification programs.
16. List and discuss the points to consider before ingesting any dietary supplements.
17. Describe the positions stands on supplements by the following organizations: AND, ACSM, IOC, NATA, CPSDA, and AASDN.

Questions

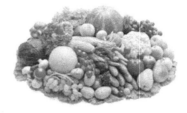

Incorporating Nutrition Programs

Performance Domain 2 - Questions
Incorporating Nutrition Programs

This domain ensures that the Nutrition Specialist has the necessary skills to implement a nutrition program in conjunction with a fitness/wellness program. This domain focuses on skills necessary to work with clients including the steps involved in implementation of an individual nutrition program; a group program; a child and teen program; a program for seniors, athletes, and vegetarians. The Nutrition Specialist must also possess the skills necessary to educate clients on sabotaging factors when it comes to maintaining health. Such factors include: why diets lead to muscle loss; inconsistencies and ambiguous labeling regulations that lead to poor food choices; eating out that also leads to poor eating choices; and other sabotaging effects such as friendly saboteurs and distortion of portion sizes, etc.

A. Prerequisites

Step 1 – Read pages 335 through 341 in the Nutrition for Professionals Textbook.

Step 2 – Answer the following questions:
1. Describe the educational requirements for successfully completing a nutrition dietetics program from an accredited university.
2. Compare and contrast the differences between a dietetics program and a master's degree program in sports nutrition.
3. List the types of state nutrition licensure laws and describe each type.
4. Provide an example of each type of licensure law and how each type affects nutrition practice in that state.
5. Explain how to choose a qualified professional to oversee a nutrition program initiated by a non-licensed professional.
6. What are the benefits of obtaining a certification in nutrition? Describe some of the factors involved when investigating certification programs.

B. *Implementing Nutrition Programs*

Step 1 – Read pages 365 through 402 in the Nutrition for Professionals Textbook.

Step 2 – Answer the following questions:
1. Explain the steps in implementing a nutrition program for individuals (interview, first appointment, requirements between appointments, second and third appointments, follow-up appointments, and details on how to end a program).
2. Which body composition measures would you use when working with individuals?
3. Explain, how you would determine the EER for a 26 year old male who weighs 237 pounds, is 6 feet 4 inches tall, and is "very active"? Explain how you would determine his BMI. What category is his BMI norm and is he at increased risk for disease?
4. Explain how you would determine the EER for a 31 year old female who weighs 132 pounds, is 5 feet 3 inches tall, and is "active". Explain how you would determine her BMI. What category is her BMI norm and is she at increased risk for disease?
5. Explain how you would go about establishing a group program.
6. How would you define and determine childhood obesity?
7. How would you establish a program for children and teens? Provide details on how you would determine caloric needs and how you would motivate children to make healthy food choices.
8. Explain how a nutrition program would differ when working with older individuals, athletes or vegetarians.

C. *Promoting Success*

Step 1 – Read pages 421 through 450 in the Nutrition for Professionals Textbook.

Step 2 – Answer the following questions:
1. Discuss the history of dieting.
2. How would you explain the AASDN Boston Beer and Prune diet to the public?
3. Why does the scale not indicate size?
4. Differentiate between the USDA labeling regulations and the FDA labeling regulations. Provide examples of each.
5. Define the following: whole grain, fat free and calorie free, organic, and gluten free.
6. Discuss the types of health claims that can be made on food labels.
7. List the types of voluntary labeling and discuss each.

8. Discuss unregulated labeling terms and the term "net carbs".

9. What role does food production and commodities play in contributing to the poor health of Americans?

10. Discuss sabotaging practices that hinder success in maintaining a healthy lifestyle.

D. Building a Successful Nutrition Business

Step 1 – Read pages 451 through 464 in the Nutrition for Professionals Textbook.

Step 2 – Answer the following questions:
1. What does Emyth refer to?

2. List factors that should be considered before starting a business (money, passion risk-taking, ethics, technology, tenacity, pros and cons).

3. List and explain the steps required in starting a business.

4. What sets you apart from others in your field that will help ensure your success?

5. What does "choosing a client base" refer to?

6. How will you price your nutrition program? Explain how you will attract sales and describe the sales process.

7. Why is it important to research your competition?

8. Does having a limited budget mean that you can't launch a successful marketing campaign? Explain your answer.

9. List the components in an advertising campaign that are essential for success and explain each component.

Questions

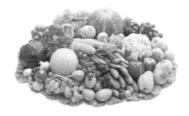

Communication /
Coaching Skills

Performance Domain 3 - Questions
Communication/Coaching Skills

Coaching and counseling are allied fields that share the goal of helping clients achieve lives of greater health and fulfillment. Both counselors and coaches help clients set measurable, attainable goals. Both teach the skills necessary for achieving the goals and both provide support and encouragement while clients work toward their goals. A major difference is the client population. Coaches work with clients who are reasonably healthy and well-functioning and wish to augment their well-being through achieving certain personal or professional goals. Goals may be specific to wellness or performance or may be more broadly aimed at achieving greater life satisfaction through, for example, changes in career or lifestyle. Coaching is focused on the present and its influence on the future. The work is also typically brief and designed to accomplish the client's goals relatively quickly. "Improvement" and "enhancement" are hallmarks of coaching. Hence, all Nutrition Specialists must acquire a working knowledge of coaching skills in order to help clients set measurable, attainable goals and teach the skills necessary for achieving those goals.

A. Coaching Skills

Step 1 – Read pages 345 through 358 in the Nutrition for Professionals Textbook.

Step 2 – Answer the following questions:
1. Define coaching.
2. What is the difference between counseling versus coaching?
3. What role does listening play in the coaching process? Explain your answer.
4. List and explain the *Stages of Readiness to Change* and its importance in the coaching process.
5. What does the "change process" refer to?. Explain your answer.
6. What is the SMART rule? What does the acronym stand for? What is the relevance of the SMART rule in coaching?
7. What does the component of "support" refer to in coaching?

Questions

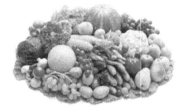

Nutrition Research /
Application and Methods

Performance Domain 4 - Questions
Nutrition Research/Application and Methods

The revolution in genetics, patent protections for bio-engineered molecules, laws strengthening intellectual property rights, and licensing and patenting of results from federally-sponsored research have created new incentives for scientists, clinicians, and academic institutions to join forces with for-profit industry in an unprecedented array of entrepreneurial activities. While many professionals are involved in research, many more read the results of research and apply it to the real world. Therefore, it is vitally important for the Nutrition Specialist to be able to critically analyze research to determine if the methods and results are valid.

A. Bias and Conflict of Interest

Step 1 – Read pages 307 through 314 in the Nutrition for Professionals Textbook.

Step 2 – Answer the following questions:
1. What is the scientific method?
2. What is bias in research? How does the scientific method minimize bias?
3. What does conflict of interest in research refer to?
4. List and describe the two types of conflicts of interest.
5. What is the Bayh-Dole Act?
6. How did the Bayh-Dole act change the research environment?
7. What is the role of government in trying to reduce conflicts of interest in research.?
8. How can conflicts of interest be managed?

B. Critical Analysis of Research

Step 1 – Read pages 315 through 327 in the Nutrition for Professionals Textbook.

Step 2 – Answer the following questions:
1. Describe the different types of study design and list the strengths and weaknesses of each design.
2. List the questions to be answered when analyzing a research paper.
3. List reputable resources for nutrition information.

Questions

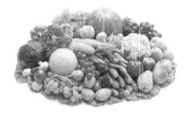

Professional and Legal Practices

Performance Domain 5 - Questions
Professional and Legal Practices

The AASDN Nutrition Specialist Certification is the only non-regulatory nutrition certification program that includes all materials used by certificants including documents and scripted programs. The AASDN Nutrition Specialist program is also the only non-regulatory nutrition certification program that includes unlimited sports dietitian support. The American Academy of Sports Dietitians and Nutritionists (AASDN) has undertaken the task of developing a more specific nutrition scope of practice for AASDN Nutrition Specialists (NS). This scope of practice is applicable to all fitness/wellness health professionals that partner with qualified, licensed professionals but is specific to AASDN certified professionals. The goal of this document is to provide AASDN certificants with clear, concise, and professional standards for inclusion of nutrition education. These guidelines are aimed at clarifying issues and adherence to all state nutrition licensure laws. Hence, this domain ensures that the AASDN Nutrition Specialist Certification program standards provide safe, effective and legal programs to the public, and that the Nutrition Specialist will continue to improve in competence in the profession through a professional code of conduct, maintain competence through continuing education, and adhere to a defined scope of practice.

A. AASDN Professional Code of Conduct

Step 1 – Read pages 21 through 28 in this study guide.

Step 2 – Answer the following questions:
1. Explain the AASDN Nutrition Specialist recertification policy.
2. What is the AASDN Nutrition Specialist renewal policy?
3. Describe the continuing education policy including contact hours and acceptable categories for contact hours.

AASDN Scope of Practice

Step 1 – Read pages 21 through 31 in this study guide.

Step 2 – Answer the following questions:
1. What is the definition of a fitness professional and wellness professional as defined in the AASDN Scope of Practice?
2. What is the definition of a medical condition as defined in the AASDN Scope of

Practice?

3. List the 10 points associated with the AASDN Code of Ethics.

4. Explain the limitations associated with the practice of nutrition for Nutrition Specialists.

5. Can a Nutrition Specialist make changes to any of the AASDN documents? Explain your answer.

6. What are the educational requirements for Nutrition Specialists?

7. Explain the AASDN standard on endorsement and sales of nutritional products.

8. Can an AASDN Nutrition Specialist sell or recommend supplements? Explain your answer.

9. What is the professional responsibility of the Nutrition Specialist with regard to boundaries of competence?

10. List the main points associated with the AASDN Professional Code of Conduct.

11. What is the AASDN policy on confidentiality?

12. What is the AASDN policy on integrity?

13. What are the actions that AASDN can take towards revocation of the AASDN Nutrition Specialist credential?

14. What is the AASDN complaint, appeals and sanctions process?

Part 3
Answers

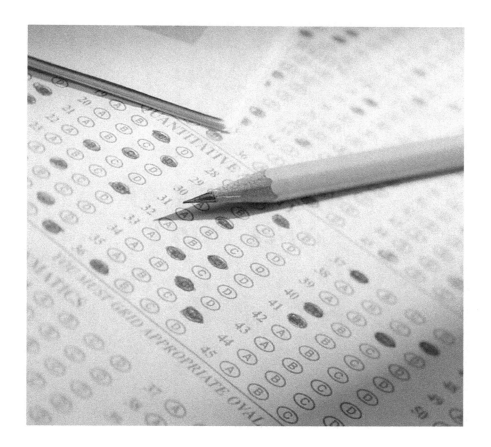

Answers

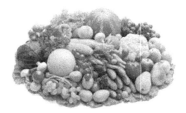

The Science of Nutrition

Performance Domain 1 - Answers
The Science of Nutrition

A. Biology of Cells

Question	Answer
1	Cells can be differentiated by whether or not they contain a nucleus.
2	A cell without a nucleus is called a prokaryotic cell and a cell with a nucleus is called a eukaryotic cell. Bacteria are examples of prokaryotes, while plant cells and animal cells are examples of eukaryotes
3	Many of the differences between plants and animals in the areas of nutrition, digestion, growth, reproduction, and defense, can be traced to the differences in cell walls. Plant cells have a rigid cell wall composed of tough fibrils of cellulose (fiber) while animal membranes are composed of lipid bilayers. Plant cells can only obtain nutrients through photosynthesis; animal cells cannot produce energy and can only obtain energy through ingestion of food.
4	Tissues include: epithelial, connective, skeletal and smooth muscle, nervous system.
5	Differences include: muscle cells have more mitochondria than fat cells (that have very few mitochondria); nerve cells and red blood cells have no mitochondria and must rely on glucose from the bloodstream for energy.

B. Nutrition Basics

Question	Answer
1	Digestion is the process by which food and drink are broken down into their smallest components so the body can absorb them to build and nourish cells and provide energy. Organs involved include: mouth, stomach, small intestines, large intestines. The digestive track consists of a series of hollow organs joined in a long, twisted tube from the mouth to the anus. Organs that make up the digestive tract are the mouth, esophagus, stomach, small intestine, large intestine (also called the colon), rectum, and anus. Inside these hollow organs is a lining called the mucosa.
2	The mucosa contains tiny glands that produce juices to help digest food. The digestive tract also contains a layer of smooth muscle that helps break down food and move it along the tract
3	Peristalsis is the wavelike muscular contractions of the GI tract that pushes its contents down the tract.
4	Absorption of most foods occurs in the small intestines. Visually, the small intestines look like a tube that has a one inch circumference. This tube extends about twenty feet and contains hundreds of folds. Because of these folds, the area of the small intestines provides a surface comparable to a quarter of a football field. The mucosa of the small intestine contains many folds that are covered with tiny finger like projections called villi. In turn, the villi are covered with microscopic projections called microvilli. The microvilli and their membranes contain hundreds of different kinds of pumps and enzymes producing tremendous specialization of absorption of nutrients. This fact combined with the large surface area allows for quick absorption of nutrients.

5	Digestive juices consist of enzymes that act on food substances causing them to break down into smaller compounds allowing these smaller compounds to be absorbed.
6	The 3 segments of the small intestines include the duodenum, the jejunum and the ileum. Specialization occurs in these segments of the small intestines. The nutrients that are ready for absorption early are absorbed near the top of the intestinal tract, those that take longer to be digested are absorbed further down the tract.
7	The vascular system (blood circulatory system) is a closed system of vessels with continuous flow of blood. The heart serves as a pump, pumping blood to all cells through arteries. Veins are vessels that carry blood to the heart and arteries are vessels that carry blood away from the heart. Arteries branch into smaller vessels known as capillaries. As the blood circulates through arteries (then capillaries), it picks up and delivers materials to the cells of the body. All cells receive oxygen and nutrients from the blood and all cells deposit carbon dioxide and other wastes into the blood. The lymphatic system is also a one- way route. Lymphatic fluid (lymph) circulates between cells of the body and collects into tiny capillary-like vessels. Lymph is almost identical to blood except that it does not contain red blood cells or platelets. Molecules in the lymphatic system collect in the thoracic duct which terminates in the subclavian vein. Contents are conducted towards the heart where they enter the circulation like other nutrients from the GI tract. One exception, however, is that nutrients entering the blood stream from the lymphatic system bypass the liver.
8	Calories are the units by which energy released from foods is measured. One kilo-calorie is the amount of heat necessary to raise the temperature of one kilogram of water one degree centigrade. While calories are listed on labels, the measurement is actually kilo-calories (10). One gram of carbohydrate equals 4 Kcal; one gram of protein also equals 4 Kcal; one gram of fat equals 9 Kcal; and one gram of alcohol equals 7 Kcal.
9	Anabolism consists of reactions in which smaller molecules are combined to build larger ones. Anabolic reactions require energy. Catabolism consists of reactions in which large molecules are broken down to smaller ones. Catabolic reactions release energy. Carbohydrates are broken down into simple sugars. Lipids consists of triglycerides, phospholipids and steroids. Triglycerides and phospholipids are broken down to fatty acids, glycerol and phosphate. Proteins are broken down to amino acids.
10	Micronutrients consists of vitamins and minerals. The body requires them in much smaller amounts than the Macronutrients.
11	Vitamins are a group of organic compounds other than protein, carbohydrates, and fats that cannot be manufactured by the body and are required in small amounts for specific functions of growth.
12	Minerals are inorganic elements essential to life that act as control agents in body reactions and cooperative factors in energy production, body building and maintenance of tissues. They retain their identity and cannot be destroyed by heat, air, acid, or mixing.
13	Homeostasis is the maintenance of constant internal conditions in body systems; i.e. balance. Examples include: glucose, pH levels, calcium, cholesterol, etc.
14	Hormones are chemical messengers secreted in trace amounts by one type of tissue. They are carried by the blood to a target tissue and they then stimulate activity in this target tissue thereby controlling metabolism.
15	Concentration of certain nutrients in certain parts of the cell also has an effect on metabolism. If too much of a product accumulates in a certain part of the cell, the increased amount of the product signals the cell to stop producing the product or transpose the product into another molecule. For example, when too much glucose enters liver cells, the excess glucose signals the cells to store glycogen.

16	Compartmentalization occurs when certain nutrients in different parts of the cell build up, and the increased amounts signal the cell to switch metabolism. For example, when fatty acids in the cytosol of the cell build up they become attached to a molecule called carnitine which carries these fatty acids into the mitochondria to be oxidized for energy. If too many fatty acids build up in the mitochondria, the extra fatty acids are then turned into a chemical called citrate. The citrate leaves the mitochondria and goes back into the cytosol where the citrate can be turned back into fatty acids.
17	The DRI's are an average daily dietary intake level sufficient to meet the nutrition requirement of nearly all (97 to 98 percent) healthy individuals in a particular life stage and gender group. There are two sets of reference values for reporting nutrients in nutrition labeling: Daily Reference Values (DRVs) and Reference Daily Intakes (RDIs). These values assist consumers in interpreting information about the amount of a nutrient that is present in a food and in comparing nutritional values of food products. DRVs are established for adults and children four or more years of age, as are RDIs, with the exception of protein. DRVs are provided for total fat, saturated fat, cholesterol, total carbohydrate, dietary fiber, sodium, potassium, and protein. RDIs are provided for vitamins and minerals and for protein for children less than four years of age and for pregnant and lactating women.
18	The intent of the Dietary Guidelines is to summarize and synthesize knowledge about individual nutrients and food components into an interrelated set of recommendations for healthy eating that can be adopted by the public. Dietary Guidelines for Americans, 2010 consists of six chapters. This first chapter introduces the document and provides information on background and purpose. The next five chapters correspond to major themes that emerged from the 2010 Dietary Guidelines for Americans review of the evidence. These recommendations are based on a preponderance of the scientific evidence for nutritional factors that are important for promoting health and lowering risk of diet-related chronic disease. Recommendations always refer to individual intake or amount rather than population average intake, unless otherwise noted. Although divided into chapters that focus on particular aspects of eating patterns, Dietary Guidelines for Americans provides integrated recommendations for health. To get the full benefit, individuals should carry out these recommendations in their entirety as part of an overall healthy eating pattern.
19	MyPyramid.gov was developed to carry the messages of the 2005 Dietary Guidelines and to make Americans aware of the vital health benefits of simple and modest improvements in nutrition, physical activity and lifestyle behavior. In 2011 MyPlate was introduced along with updating of the USDA food patterns for the 2010 Dietary Guidelines for Americans.
20	The Healthy Eating Plate is based on the best available science and was not subjected to political and commercial pressures from food industry lobbyists.

C. Carbohydrates

Question	Answer
1	See Nutrition for Professionals Textbook page 35 for a discussion on the process of carbohydrate digestion.
2	Absorption of carbohydrates occurs when the monosaccharides are absorbed into the small intestinal cells. They cross the small intestinal cells and are washed into the bloodstream by a rush of circulating blood which carries them to the liver.
3	The monosaccharides are delivered through the bloodstream to the liver where the liver converts them to glucose. There are five possible fates for glucose in the liver: glucose can be converted into glycogen; glucose can be used for energy by liver cells; any

	amount beyond that which can be stored as carbohydrate will be turned into fatty acids, which in turn can travel to the fat cells and be stored as fat; the liver can add a phosphate group to glucose and store it as glucose-6-phosphate (discussed in more detail in Chapter 5); glucose can also be made into nucleotides.
4	Glycogen is a highly branched polysaccharide consisting of links of glucose molecules. Immediately upon entry into cells, glucose combines with phosphate, a process known as phosphorylation. The phosphorylation of glucose is irreversible in most cells except in liver cells, renal tubular cells, and intestinal epithelial cells. These cells contain the enzyme glucose phosphatase which catalyzes the reverse reaction know as glycogenolysis (the breakdown of glycogen to glucose). In other words, only liver cells, renal tubular cells and intestinal epithelial cells have the ability to catabolize glycogen to glucose. Muscle cells lack the enzyme glucose phosphatase, which is required to release glucose into the blood, so the glycogen stored in muscle is for internal use only and cannot be shared with other cells. Muscle cells can store more glycogen than liver cells. For example, the average 150 pound male can store approximately 1800 calories of carbohydrate, 1400 calories in muscle in the form of glycogen, 320 calories in the liver in the form of glycogen, and approximately 80 calories of glucose in the bloodstream.
5	See Nutrition for Professionals Textbook page 37 and 38 for a discussion on glucose homeostasis including the hormones involved.
6	Certain cells of the body do not have insulin receptors and are referred to as non-insulin-dependent cells. Most cells of the body are insulin-dependent cells with the exception of red blood cells, nerve cells, brain cells, and a variety of cells involved in vision. These non-insulin-dependent cells are quite different in that insulin has either little or no effect on glucose utilization or uptake. Another distinguishing factor is that these cells (red blood cells, nerve cells, cells involved in vision, etc.) can only use glucose as an energy source. Therefore, prevention of damage to these cells requires glucose levels to be maintained within the homeostatic range.
7	The glucose time curve refers to a finite amount of glycogen that can be stored in the body and the processes that occur when glycogen stores are depleted.
8	See Nutrition for Professionals Textbook page 39 for details concerning the process of gluconeogenesis and its role in glucose homeostasis.
9	Ketosis is a metabolic state that occurs when the liver converts fat into fatty acids and ketone bodies. Ketones, acetoacetate and β-hydroxybutyrate, are small carbon fragments that are the fuel created by the breakdown of fat stores. Biochemically, ketones closely resemble glucose. Some cells (such as muscle cells) can switch to utilization of ketones for energy, while the non-insulin dependent cells previously discussed (brain cells, nerve cells, etc.) cannot. With the use of ketones by muscle cells and other cells, the body can survive weeks and even months. Note: ketosis is always accompanied by the catabolism of amino acids.
10	Absorption rates of carbohydrates differ depending on several factors. Simple sugars in the absence of nutrients such as fiber, fat, and protein are absorbed quickly and enter the bloodstream quickly. When complex carbohydrates (legumes, breads, etc.) are absorbed in the presence of other nutrients such as fat, protein, or fiber, the absorption rate of the sugar is decreased (slowed). In this circumstance large amounts of simple sugars do not flood the bloodstream and the body is not forced to form triglycerides.
11	The glycemic response refers to how quickly glucose is absorbed after a person eats, how high blood glucose rises, and how quickly it returns to normal.
12	Different foods elicit different glycemic responses, and the glycemic index classifies foods according to this response.
13	Glycemic load is a similar concept to glycemic index; however, glycemic load scores a food product based on both carbohydrate content and portion size. A food's glycemic load is determined by multiplying its glycemic index by the amount of carbohydrate it

	contains. In general, a glycemic load of 20 or more is high, 11 to 19 is medium, and 10 or under is low.
14	Insulin resistance, or metabolic syndrome, describes a combination of health problems that have a common link, i.e., an increased risk of diabetes and early heart disease. Diseases or conditions associated with insulin resistance include the following: obesity, Type 2 diabetes, high blood pressure, abnormal cholesterol levels, heart disease, and polycystic ovary syndrome. People with this syndrome have high levels of insulin in the blood as a marker of the disease rather than a cause. Over time people with insulin resistance can develop prediabetes or diabetes as the high insulin levels can no longer compensate for elevated sugars. The signs of insulin resistance syndrome include impaired fasting blood sugar, impaired glucose tolerance, or type 2 diabetes which occurs because the pancreas is unable to turn out enough insulin to overcome the insulin resistance. Blood sugar levels rise and prediabetes or diabetes is diagnosed. High blood pressure has been associated with insulin resistance. The mechanism is unclear, but studies suggest that the higher the blood pressure, the higher the insulin resistance. The typical cholesterol levels of a person with insulin resistance are low HDL, or good cholesterol, and high levels of triglycerides. Insulin resistance can result in atherosclerosis (hardening of the arteries) and an increased risk of blood clots. A major factor in the development of insulin resistance syndrome is obesity, especially abdominal obesity or belly fat. While obesity promotes insulin resistance, weight loss can improve the body's ability to recognize and use insulin appropriately. Protein in the urine, a sign that kidney damage has occurred, is associated with insulin resistance, although not everyone uses this component to define the syndrome.
15	There is no simple test to diagnose or treat insulin resistance syndrome. Rather, a physician may suspect the syndrome if any of the following are present: A waist size of 40 inches or more in men and 35 inches or more in women; Increased levels of triglycerides (a type of fat in the blood); Low HDL, or "good," cholesterol level (Less than 40 mg/dL for men and 50 mg/dL for women); High blood pressure of 130/85 or higher, or being treated for high blood pressure; Fasting blood glucose levels of 100 mg/dL or above, or being treated for diabetes.
16	Dietary fiber consists of nondigestible carbohydrates and lignin that are intrinsic and intact in plants; functional fiber is defined as isolated, nondigestible carbohydrates that have beneficial physiologic effects in humans. The recommended intake for males under 50 years old is 38 grams per day, and for males over 50 years old, 30 grams per day. For females under 50 years old the recommended intake is 30 grams per day and 21 grams per day for females under 50 years old. Diets rich in fibrous foods, such as whole grains, legumes, vegetables, and fruits, may protect against heart attack and stroke by lowering blood pressure, improving blood lipids, and reducing inflammation (the immune system's response to infection or injury). High fiber foods also play a key role in managing and preventing diabetes. In people with diabetes, fiber, particularly soluble fiber, can slow the absorption of sugar and help improve blood sugar levels. Another benefit attributed to dietary fiber is prevention of colorectal cancer. Fibers may help prevent colon cancer by diluting, binding, and rapidly removing potential cancer-causing agents from the colon. Dietary fibers also enhance the health of the large intestine. Large, soft stools ease elimination and reduce pressure in the lower bowel, preventing constipation and making it less likely that hemorrhoids will form.
17	See Nutrition for Professionals Textbook pages 49,50, 51 for a discussion on alcohol.
18	The most common approach to classifying sweeteners groups them as nutritive and nonnutritive sweeteners. Nutritive sweeteners contain carbohydrate and provide energy; they include sugars, caloric sweeteners, and added sugars. Sugars occur naturally in fruit, vegetables, and dairy products. They are also added to foods in processing or cooking. Nonnutritive sweeteners provide little or no calories when ingested. They are referred to as high intensity sweeteners since they are many times sweeter than sugar. See Nutrition for Professionals Textbook pages 51 through 56 for further discussion on sweeteners.

D. Lipids

Question	Answer
1	Fats refers to a subcategory of nutrients known as lipids. Although the words "oils", "fats", and "lipids" are all used to refer to fats, in reality, fat is a subset of lipid. "Oils" is usually used to refer to lipids that are liquid at normal room temperature, while "fats" is usually used to refer to lipids that are solid at normal room temperature. "Lipids" is used to refer to both liquid and solid fats, along with other related substances. The word "oil" is also used for any substance that does not mix with water and has a greasy feel, such as petroleum (or crude oil), heating oil, and essential oils, regardless of its chemical structure.
2	Triglycerides consist of a glycerol molecule and three fatty acids. Glycerol is an alcohol composed of a three carbon chain that serves as the backbone of the triglyceride molecule. Most of the stored fat in the body is triglyceride and they are the principal storage forms of energy in the human body. They also form a layer of fat under the skin for insulation and surround organs to protect against shock and injury. A phospholipid has a glycerol molecule and two fatty acids. The third fatty acid is replaced by a phosphate group. The phosphate group mixes with water while the fatty acid portion mixes with fat. The phosphate group attached to phospholipids is polar and water-soluble, while its fatty acids are oil-soluble. The phospholipids spread out in a thin layer over surfaces of water and form double-layered membranes that surround every living cell of all living organisms. See Nutrition for Professionals Textbook pages 69 and 70 for a discussion on the roles of each.
3	Saturated fatty acids are the simplest of the fatty acids. They have no double bonds between the carbon atoms of the fatty acid chain; hence, they are fully saturated with hydrogen atoms. An unsaturated fatty acid contains one or more double bonds in the fatty acid chain. A fat molecule is monounsaturated if it contains one double bond and polyunsaturated if it contains more than one double bond. Double bonds in unsaturated fatty acids may be in either a *cis* or *trans* isomer, depending on the geometry of the double bond. In the *cis* conformation, hydrogens are on the same side of the double bond; whereas in the *trans* conformation, they are on opposite sides. Natural sources of fatty acids are rich in the cis isomer; whereas hydrogenated products are rich in the trans isomer.
4	In the trans configuration, the hydrogen atoms on the carbons involved in the double bond are on opposite sides of the molecule. This configuration removes the "kink" or bend in the molecule and produces the trans isomer. The molecule now has the same straight configuration as saturated fatty acids, and hence produces many of the same arterial damaging effects as saturated fatty acids. Trans fatty acids are formed when hydrogen is added to unsaturated fats. Trans fatty acids occur from natural sources and are commercially produced. Low quantities of trans fatty acids in food products are derived from ruminant animals, mostly dairy products and meats.
5	Two unsaturated fatty acids are essential; linoleic and linolenic acid. They are deemed essential because the body cannot make them and they are required; hence, they must be obtained from food for life to be sustained. See Nutrition for Professionals Textbook pages 74 and 75 for a discussion on requirements.
6	Essential fatty acids are precursors to hormone-like substances called eicosanoids. Eicosanoids exert important effects on the immune system, cardiovascular system, reproductive system and central nervous system. All cells can form eicosanoids, but tissues differ in enzyme profile and hence in the products they can form.
7	Prostaglandins are similar to hormones in that they act as chemical messengers, but they do not move to other sites and they work within the cells where they are synthesize. A diversity of receptors means that prostaglandins act on many types of cells and have a wide variety of effects. A major effect of prostaglandins is control of platelet aggregation.

	See Nutrition for Professionals Textbook page 77 for details concerning the 3 types of prostaglandins.
8	Research indicates that there are many beneficial effects of omega-3 fatty acids. Regular consumption helps prevent irregular heartbeat and blood clots, improves lipid profile, lowers blood pressure, supports a healthy immune system, and suppresses inflammation.
9	Nearly all fish and shellfish contain traces of mercury. For most people, the risk from mercury by eating fish and shellfish is not a health concern. The risks from mercury in fish and shellfish depend on the amount of fish and shellfish eaten and the levels of mercury in the fish and shellfish. Some fish and shellfish contain higher levels of mercury that may harm an unborn baby or a young child's developing nervous system. The Food and Drug Administration (FDA) and the Environmental Protection Agency (EPA) are advising women who may become pregnant, pregnant women, nursing mothers, and young children to avoid some types of fish and eat fish and shellfish that are lower in mercury. By following the four recommendations listed below for selecting and eating fish or shellfish, consumers can reduce their exposure to the harmful effects of mercury: • Do not eat shark, swordfish, king mackerel, or tilefish because they contain high levels of mercury. • Eat up to 12 ounces (four 3 ounce servings) a week of a variety of fish and shellfish that are lower in mercury. • Five of the most commonly eaten fish that are low in mercury are shrimp, canned light tuna, salmon, pollock, and catfish. Another commonly eaten fish, albacore ("white") tuna has more mercury than canned light tuna. Fish consumption appears to be the major pathway of exposure to PCB. The FDA required limits of PCBs include 0.2 parts per million (ppm) in infant and junior foods, 0.3 ppm in eggs, 1.5 ppm in milk and other dairy products (fat basis), 2 ppm in fish and shellfish (edible portions), and 3 ppm in poultry and red meat (fat basis).
10	Steroids are organic compounds derived from 17 carbon atoms composed of four rings. There are hundreds of different types of steroids in plants, animals, and fungi, and they are involved in a variety of physiological processes. Examples of steroids include the dietary fat cholesterol, and the sex hormones estradiol and testosterone. Cholesterol is required to build and maintain membranes; it modulates membrane fluidity over the range of physiological temperatures. In the liver, cholesterol is converted to bile, which is then stored in the gallbladder. Bile contains bile salts, which solubilize fats in the digestive tract and aids in the intestinal absorption of fat molecules, as well as fat-soluble vitamins, A, D, E, K. Cholesterol is an important precursor molecule for the synthesis of vitamin D and the steroid hormones, including the adrenal gland hormones cortisol and aldosterone, as well as the sex hormones progesterone, estrogens, and testosterone, and their derivatives.
11	See Nutrition for Professionals Textbook pages 81 and 82 for a discussion of digestion of fats into their constituent components.
12	Emulsified fats, not the bile acids, are absorbed into the cells of the small intestine. Emulsified fats include monoglycerides, fatty acids, glycerol, fat soluble vitamins and cholesterol (side chains removed). To reiterate, the fatty acid on the middle position of the triglyceride (mono and polyunsaturated fatty acids with lower melting points) is easily absorbed as a monoglyceride even if normally poorly absorbed when present as a free fatty acid. This mechanism assures greater absorption of the essential fatty acids which are preferentially attached to the number two position. Once absorbed, the fats must be reassembled to be transported throughout the body.
13	See Nutrition for Professionals Textbook pages 82 and 83 for details concerning the transport of fat including the exogenous and endogenous pathways.

E. Proteins

Question	Answer
1	Proteins are linear, large organic molecules built from 20 different amino acids. The extraordinary structure of proteins enables them to play more versatile roles in the body than carbohydrates or lipids. Proteins are classified according to their structure. Some proteins are large globular compounds and are found in tissue fluids. Enzymes, protein hormones, hemoglobin, myoglobin, globulins and albumins of blood are all globular proteins. Other proteins form long chains bound together in a parallel fashion, and are called fibrous proteins. These consist of long, folded chains of amino acids and are the proteins of connective tissue and elastic tissue including collagen, elastin, and keratin. See Nutrition for Professionals Textbook pages 95 and 96 for more details on roles of proteins.
2	Twenty amino acids are biosynthesized from other molecules, but organisms differ in which ones they can synthesize and which ones must be provided in their diet. The ones that cannot be synthesized by an organism, but required, are called essential amino acids. Besides being the building blocks for proteins, amino acids have other vital roles as well. Many amino acids are used to synthesize other molecules, for example: gamma-aminobutyric acid, and glutamate are neurotransmitters; tryptophan is a precursor of the neurotransmitter serotonin and the vitamin niacin; glycine is a neurotransmitter and a precursor of porphyrins such as heme; arginine is a precursor of nitric oxide; carnitine is used in lipid transport within the cell; ornithine and S-adenosylmethionine are precursors of polyamines; homocysteine is an intermediate in S-adenosylmethionine recycling; tyrosine serves as a precursor for norepinephrine and epinephrine. Tyrosine can also make the pigment melanin. A small group of amino acids comprised of isoleucine, phenylalanine, threonine, tryptophan, and tyrosine give rise to both glucose and fatty acid precursors and are thus characterized as being glucogenic and ketogenic.
3	Non essential amino acids are not required in the diet because the body can synthesize them from essential amino acids. See the Nutrition for Professionals Textbook page 98 for a list of non essential amino acids.
4	There are nine essential amino acids (also known as indispensable amino acids) that the body cannot synthesize or synthesize in sufficient amounts to meet the needs of the body. A third class, known as the conditionally essential amino acids are synthesized from other amino acids. See the Nutrition for Professionals Textbook page 98 for a list of essential amino acids.
5	Alanine (a non essential amino acid) along with glutamine, is an interorgan nitrogen carrier and an energy producing amino acid. Alanine plays a key role in the glucose–alanine cycle between tissues and liver. When glucose is unavailable, muscle and other tissues degrade amino acids for fuel. Amino groups are transaminated to form glutamate. Glutamate can then transfer its amino group to pyruvate, forming alanine and alpha-ketoglutarate. The alanine formed passes into the blood and is transported to the liver. A reverse of the reaction takes place in the liver in which alanine is transaminated into glutamate forming glucose (through gluconeogenesis) and the glucose formed is released through the circulation system. Glutamate in the liver enters mitochondria and degrades into ammonium which in turn participates in the urea cycle to form urea.
6	Nitrogen is a chemical element that has the symbol N and atomic number 7 and atomic weight of 14. Elemental nitrogen is a colorless, odorless, tasteless and mostly inert diatomic gas at standard conditions, constituting 78.1% by volume of Earth's atmosphere. Nitrogen is present in all living organisms in proteins, nucleic acids, and other molecules. Nitrogen cannot be "fixed" (produced) by humans and must be obtained through absorption of amino acids.

7	Nitrogen cannot be "fixed" (produced) by humans and must be obtained through absorption of amino acids. Without nitrogen amino acids, nucleic acids and other essential molecules cannot be synthesized. Nitrogen is toxic to cells and must be eliminated daily. The liver is the major site of nitrogen metabolism in the body. In times of dietary surplus, the potentially toxic nitrogen of amino acids is eliminated via transamination, deamination, and urea formation. The carbon skeletons are generally conserved as carbohydrate, via gluconeogenesis, or as fatty acid via fatty acid synthesis pathways. In fevers, fasting, and wasting diseases there is a net loss of nitrogen from the body.
8	Amino acids fall into three categories: glucogenic, ketogenic, or both glucogenic and ketogenic. Glucogenic amino acids are those that give rise to a net production of pyruvate or energy cycle intermediates, all of which are precursors to glucose via gluconeogenesis. All amino acids except lysine and leucine are at least partly glucogenic. Lysine and leucine are the only amino acids that are solely ketogenic, neither of which can bring about net glucose production
9	See Nutrition for Professionals Textbook pages 100 and 101 for a description of digestion of proteins.
10	The role of dietary proteins is to provide the body with amino acids that the body can use to synthesize its own proteins. A misconception is that proteins in the diet can affect protein synthesis in the body. As previously mentioned, all dietary proteins are digested into amino acids. Once a protein is denatured it no longer functions as a protein but rather is reduced to chains of amino acids. Once absorbed, all amino acids may be used for energy or synthesized into needed compounds, hence proteins in the diet cannot affect protein synthesis in the body. The role of dietary proteins is to provide the body with the necessary building blocks (essential amino acids) needed by the body to synthesize the required proteins. Another misconception is that eating predigested proteins (amino acid supplements) saves the body from having to digest proteins. This is not the case. The digestion system handles whole proteins in a more efficient manner than predigested amino acids because it dismantles and absorbs the amino acids at a rate that is optimal for absorption.
11	Free amino acids and dipeptides (sometimes tripeptides) are absorbed into the intestinal cells. In the small intestine, carrier molecules transport these amino acids and small peptides across the intestinal cells, into the bloodstream, and into the body. Once in the bloodstream, amino acids enter cells by transporters.
12	See Nutrition for Professionals Textbook pages 101 and 102 for a description of amino acid transport systems and the role of the blood-brain barrier in control of the CNS.
13	See Nutrition for Professionals Textbook pages 102 through 106. for a description of the methods for determining protein quality. PDCAAS are currently being used; however, the use of DIAAS are being recommended.

F. Energy

Question	Answer
1	Energy production consists of four phases: ATP-PC, Glycolysis, Tricarboxylic acid (TCA) cycle, Electron transport chain. See Nutrition for Professionals Textbook pages 117 through 119 for details concerning each phase.
2	See Nutrition for Professionals Textbook pages 119 through 127 for factors involved in energy nutrient utilization.
3	See Nutrition for Professionals Textbook pages 127 through 131 for the percentages/grams energy nutrient intake as defined by the DRI, AND, ACSM, and the IOC.

4	The Dietary Reference Intake (DRI) for water for males is 3.7 liters (125.1 ounces) per day and 2.7 liters (91.3 ounces) per day for females. Sources include all beverages including water and moisture in foods. High moisture foods include most fruits, and soups.
5	See Nutrition for Professionals Textbook pages 131 through 134 for a discussion on nutrient timing and the recommendations by the AND, ACSM, and the IOC.
6	The AND and ACSM recommend no additional vitamin and mineral supplementation if an athlete obtains sufficient energy from a wide variety of foods. Supplementation may be individually prescribed by the attending healthcare professional for certain athletes, such as those restricting energy intake, vegetarians, people who are ill, recovering from injury, or with specific medical conditions. Vegetarians may require vitamin B12, iron, calcium, vitamin D, riboflavin, and zinc supplementation. Research has indicated that possible supplementation with antioxidants might be warranted. The IOC position supports the AND and ACSM conclusion that energy requirements be met through dietary means, and additional supplementation is not warranted. Toxic levels may impair muscle functioning and reduce training adaptations to exercise. The IOC also cautions against the use of single-nutrient, high-dose antioxidant supplements.
7	The 3 components for determining total energy requirements include basal metabolic rate; thermal effect of food; and physical activity. See Nutrition for Professionals Textbook pages 134 and 135 for details concerning each.
8	Men 19 Years and Older EER = [662 – (9.53 x Age)] + PA X [(15.91 x Weight) + (539.6 x Height)] Women 19 Years and Older EER = [354 – (6.91 x Age)] + PA X [(9.36 x Weight) + (726 x Height)]
9	In working with children (up to 16 years of age), the EER tends to over estimate total caloric needs for children. Another method from the Institute of Medicine (IOM) utilizes information taken from the IOM Dietary Reference Intakes report, 2002, which utilizes "Reference size," as determined by IOM. Reference size is based on median height and weight for children ages up to age 18 years of age.
10	The BMR component of EER does not take into account body composition, which includes the percentages of lean body mass and fat in the body. Muscle burns many more calories than fat. Leaner bodies need more calories than bodies that are less lean. Hence, a person with an above average amount of muscle will have a higher BMR than calculated and therefore a higher EER; and a person with a below average amount of muscle will have a lower BMR than calculated and therefore a lower EER (54,57). The "ideal" lean body mass is based on the ideal body fat percentage of 15% for men and 22% for women.

G. Nutrition and Disease

Question	Answer
1	Diabetes is a disease in which the body does not produce or properly use insulin. It is associated with long-term complications that affect almost every part of the body. In the first stage of diabetes, cells require energy because glucose cannot enter insulin dependent cells. The build up of sugar in the blood can cause an increase in urination by signaling the kidneys to release glucose through the urine, which can lead to large amounts of fluid losses causing dehydration. When a person with type 2 diabetes becomes severely dehydrated and is not able to drink enough fluids to make up for the fluid losses, they may develop life-threatening complications. As the disease progresses, the high glucose levels in the blood damage red blood cells, nerve cells, cells involved in vision, kidney cells, and heart cells.

2	Type 1 diabetes is an autoimmune disease usually diagnosed in children and young adults, and was previously known as juvenile diabetes. In type 1 diabetes, the immune system attacks the insulin-producing beta cells in the pancreas and destroys them. The pancreas then produces little or no insulin, thus requiring administration of exogenous insulin several times per day or via an insulin pump. In type 2 diabetes, either the body does not produce enough insulin or the cells ignore the insulin. When type 2 diabetes is diagnosed, the pancreas is usually producing enough insulin, but for unknown reasons, the body cannot use the insulin effectively, a condition called insulin resistance. Gestational diabetes develops only during pregnancy.
3	The fasting plasma glucose test is the preferred test for diagnosing type 1 or type 2 diabetes. An oral glucose tolerance test is taken in a laboratory or the doctor's office and measures plasma glucose at timed intervals over a 3-hour period.
4	See Nutrition for Professionals Textbook pages 154 through 156 for 50 ways to reduce diabetes risk.
5	Physical activity can lower blood glucose levels rapidly. In diabetic patients, regular activity favorably affects the body's ability to use insulin to control glucose levels in the blood. Although the effect of an exercise program on any single risk factor may generally be small, the effect of continued, moderate exercise on overall cardiovascular risk, when combined with other lifestyle modifications (such as proper nutrition, smoking cessation, and medication use), can be dramatic.
6	Cardiovascular disease refers to the class of diseases that involve the heart or blood vessels (arteries and veins). While the term technically refers to any disease that affects the cardiovascular system, it is usually used to refer to those related to atherosclerosis (arterial disease).Some of the risk factors for CV disease include: age, gender, high blood pressure, high serum cholesterol levels, tobacco smoking, alcohol consumption, family history, obesity, lack of physical activity, psychosocial factors, diabetes, air pollution.
7	Some of the same factors are involved in heart disease including diabetes and kidney failure, overweight and obesity, poor diet, physical inactivity and excessive alcohol use.
8	Lowering blood pressure and cholesterol are the largest factors in reducing risk of heart disease. Currently practiced measures to prevent cardiovascular disease include: Eat a low saturated fat, high-fiber diet including whole grains and plenty of fresh fruits and vegetables (at least five portions per day); cease tobacco use and avoid second-hand smoke; limit alcohol consumption to the recommended daily limits consumption of 1-2 standard alcoholic drinks per day; lower blood pressures, if elevated; decrease body fat (BMI); increase daily activity to 30 minutes of vigorous exercise per day at least five times per week; decrease psychosocial stress. If these measures don't work a physician may recommend cholesterol lowering medications.
9	Atherosclerosis is a condition in which an artery wall thickens as a result of the accumulation of fatty materials. It is a chronic inflammatory response in the walls of arteries, caused largely by the accumulation of macrophage white blood cells, and promoted by low-density lipoproteins, with inadequate removal of fats and cholesterol from the macrophages by high-density lipoproteins. Atherosclerosis usually begins with the accumulation of soft fatty streaks along the inner arterial walls, especially at branch points. Ruptures expose thrombogenic material, such as collagen, to the circulation and eventually induce thrombus (clot) formation in the lumen. Upon formation, intraluminal thrombi can occlude (obstruct) arteries outright (i.e. coronary occlusion), but more often they detach, move into the circulation, and eventually occlude or obstruct smaller downstream branches causing thromboembolism.
10	See Nutrition for Professionals Textbook pages 159 for table listing levels of cholesterol, HDL and LDL associated with increased risk for CV disease.
11	See Nutrition for Professionals Textbook pages 160 through 161 for a discussion on cholesterol lowering medications.

12	See Nutrition for Professionals Textbook pages 161 for a list of other ways to reduce cholesterol levels.
13	See Nutrition for Professionals Textbook pages 162 through 165 for details concerning other factors involved in CV disease risk including L-carnitine, homocysteine, high sensitivity c-reactive protein, and coronary calcium scan.
14	A sedentary lifestyle is one of the 5 major risk factors for cardiovascular disease. Evidence from many scientific studies shows that reducing these risk factors decreases the chance of having a heart attack or experiencing another cardiac event and reduces the possibility of needing a coronary procedure (bypass surgery or coronary angioplasty). Regular exercise has a favorable effect on many of the established risk factors for cardiovascular disease. For example, exercise promotes weight reduction and can help reduce blood pressure. Exercise can reduce cholesterol levels in the blood, as well as total cholesterol, and can raise the HDL level.
15	Hypertension is a chronic medical condition in which the blood pressure in the arteries is elevated. This requires the heart to work harder than normal to circulate blood through the blood vessels. Normal blood pressure at rest is within the range of 80-120mmHg systolic (top reading) and 60-90mmHg diastolic (bottom reading). High blood pressure is said to be present if it is persistently at or above 140/90 mm Hg.
16	See Nutrition for Professionals Textbook pages 166 through 168 for a discussion on the dash diets and the Mediterranean diet.
17	Epidemiological studies indicate that the relationship between sedentary behavior and hypertension is so strong that the National Heart Foundation , the World Health Organization and International Society of Hypertension, the United States Joint National Committee on Detection, Evaluation and Treatment of High Blood Pressure, and the American College of Sports Medicine (ACSM) have all recommended increased physical activity as a first line intervention for preventing and treating patients with prehypertension and hypertension. See Nutrition for Professionals Textbook pages 168 through 169 for further discussion.
18	A stroke occurs when a clot blocks the blood supply to part of the brain or when a blood vessel in or around the brain bursts. In either case, parts of the brain become damaged.
19	Factors in developing stroke that cannot be modified include: age, race, gender, family history of stroke. Factors that can be modified include: hypertension, smoking, heart disease, know the warning signs of stroke, diabetes, cholesterol imbalance, physical inactivity and obesity.
20	The warning signs of stroke include: sudden numbness or weakness of face, arm, or leg, especially on one side of the body; sudden confusion, or trouble talking or understanding speech; sudden trouble seeing in one or both eyes; sudden trouble walking, dizziness, or loss of balance or coordination; sudden severe headache with no known cause. Other danger signs that may occur include double vision, drowsiness, and nausea or vomiting.
21	Regular physical activity to reduce the risk of stroke is similar to that of heart disease. Regular physical activity can improve heart and lung function, raise HDL and lower triglycerides. The American Heart Association recommends 30 minutes of moderately intense aerobic activity at least 5 days per week or 25 minutes of vigorous aerobic activity at least three days per week and moderate to high intensity muscle strengthening activity at least two or more days per week.
22	Cancers that maybe affected by lifestyle, diet and exercise include: all cancers caused by smoking and heavy use of alcohol; one third of new cancer cases will be attributed to overweight, obesity, physical inactivity, and poor nutrition. Certain cancers can be prevented through behavioral changes: human papillomavirus (HPV), hepatitis B virus (HBV), hepatitis C virus (HCV), human immunodeficiency virus (HIV), and Helicobacter pylori (H. pylori). Regular screenings and early detection can reduce cancer risk and severity.

23	Celiac disease is a chronic inflammatory condition caused by ingestion of dietary gluten (a protein found in wheat, barley, and rye). The diagnosis relies on the clinical picture of the patient, serological markers, characteristic findings of small intestinal biopsy, and clinical improvement on a gluten-free diet. A gluten-free diet is the only current treatment.
24	GI disorders generally fall into two categories — functional and inflammatory. Inflammatory bowel disease is a group of inflammatory conditions of the colon and small intestine. Irritable bowel syndrome is a disorder that leads to abdominal pain and cramping, changes in bowel movements, and other symptoms. Irritable bowel syndrome is not the same as inflammatory bowel disease, which includes Crohn's disease and ulcerative colitis. In IBS, the structure of the bowel is not abnormal.
25	The major types of inflammatory bowel disease are Crohn's disease and ulcerative colitis. Crohn's disease is a type of inflammatory bowel disease that may affect any part of the gastrointestinal tract from mouth to anus, causing a wide variety of symptoms. Because the symptoms of Crohn's disease are similar to other intestinal disorders, such as irritable bowel syndrome and ulcerative colitis, it can be difficult to diagnose. Ulcerative colitis causes inflammation and ulcers in the top layer of the lining of the large intestine. In Crohn's disease, all layers of the intestine may be involved, and normal healthy bowel can be found between sections of diseased bowel.
26	Gastroesophageal reflux disease, or GERD, is a chronic condition in which the lower esophageal sphincter allows gastric acids to reflux into the esophagus, causing heartburn, acid indigestion, and possible injury to the esophageal lining. Various methods to treat the disease range from lifestyle measures to the use of medication or surgical procedures. It is essential for individuals who suffer persistent heartburn or other chronic and recurrent symptoms to seek an accurate diagnosis and work with their physician, and to receive the most effective treatment available. In general, sufferers of GERD should decrease citrus, chocolate, caffeine, mints, spicy foods, fried foods, high fat foods. Other lifestyle changes include: exercise, weight loss if necessary, wear loose fitting clothing, and elevating the head of the bed may help decrease symptoms.
27	CKD is diagnosed through scans, biopsies, and urine and laboratory testing. CKD presents in 5 stages which correlate with a glomerular filtration rate (GFR) or percent kidney function based on blood creatintine levels, age, race and gender. A person with normal kidney function can have a GFR or 90-100+ percent. See table in Nutrition for Professionals Textbook, page 180 for abnormal levels.
28	See Nutrition for Professionals Textbook page 180 for a description of the stages of kidney failure.
29	See Nutrition for Professionals Textbook pages 180 and 181 for a description of the dietary changes required to compensate for the reduced excretion of certain nutrients in kidney failure.

H. Vitamins and Minerals

Question	Answer
1	The water soluble vitamins include the B vitamins and Vitamin C. See Nutrition for Professionals Textbook page 199 through 206 for details concerning metabolic roles, foods, recommended intakes, deficiency and toxicity, for each vitamin.
2	The fat soluble vitamins include Vitamin A, D, E, and K. See Nutrition for Professionals Textbook page 206 through 215 for details concerning metabolic roles, foods, recommended intakes, deficiency and toxicity, for each vitamin.
3	See Nutrition for Professionals Textbook pages 228 and 229 for a discussion on the importance of water and recommended intake, deficiency and toxicity symptoms.

4	The major minerals include calcium, sodium, chloride, potassium, sulfur, phosphorous, and magnesium. See Nutrition for Professionals Textbook pages 230 through 238 for details concerning each major mineral.
5	The trace minerals include iron, zinc, iodine, selenium, copper, manganese, fluoride, chromium, and molybdenum. See Nutrition for Professionals Textbook pages 238 through 249 for details concerning each trace mineral.

I. Complimentary and Alternative Medicine

Question	Answer
1	When describing non-mainstream health approaches people often use the words "alternative" and "complementary" interchangeably, but the two terms refer to different concepts: "Complementary" generally refers to using a non-mainstream approach together with conventional medicine; "Alternative" refers to using a non-mainstream approach in place of conventional medicine. True alternative medicine is not common.
2	The National Center for Complementary and Alternative Medicine (NCCAM) is the Federal Government's lead agency for scientific research on complementary and alternative medicine (CAM).The mission of NCCAM is to explore complementary and alternative healing practices in the context of rigorous science, train CAM researchers, and disseminate authoritative information to the public and professionals.
3	NCCAM generally uses the term "complementary health approaches" when discussing the practices and products they research. NCCAM categorizes complementary health approaches into two subgroups – dietary supplements and mind body practices. Some approaches may not neatly fit into either of these groups—for example, the practices of traditional healers, Ayurveda medicine from India, traditional Chinese medicine, homeopathy, and naturopathy.
4	Dietary supplements includes a variety of products, such as herbs (subcategory of botanicals), vitamins and minerals, amino acids, enzymes, and/or other ingredients. Before 1994, the original definition of a supplement was a product that contained one or more of the essential nutrients. After DSHEA, the definition of a supplement was changed to any product intended for ingestion as a supplement to the diet. This definition now includes liquid, pill, capsule, or tablet forms of vitamins, minerals, herbs, botanicals and other plant derived substances, amino acids and concentrates, metabolites, constituents, and extracts of these substances.
5	Mind and body practices include a large and diverse group of procedures including acupuncture, massage therapy, meditation, spinal manipulation, Tai chi and qi gong, yoga, healing touch, and hypnotherapy.
6	A major reason for the explosion in the use of dietary supplements is the passage of the Dietary Supplement Health and Education Act of 1994 (DSHEA) by Congress. Before 1994, The Food and Drug Administration regulated dietary supplements to ensure that they were safe and wholesome and that their labeling was truthful and not misleading. The Dietary Supplement Health and Education Act of 1994 (Public Law 103-417, DSHEA), authorized the establishment of the Office of Dietary Supplements (ODS) at the National Institute of Health (NIH).
7	After the passage of DSHEA the definition of a supplement changed (see answer 4). Under DSHEA, Congress amended the Federal Food, Drug, and Cosmetic Act (FD&C Act) to include provisions that apply only to dietary supplements and dietary ingredients of dietary supplements. As a result of these provisions, dietary ingredients used in dietary supplements are no longer subject to the premarket safety evaluations required of other new food ingredients or for new uses of old food ingredients. The FDA notes that under the DSHEA supplements are no longer regulated like other products such as drugs, additives, cosmetics, foods (animal and human), medical

	devices, and radiation emitting consumer products (microwaves).
8	The Dietary Supplement Health and Education Act of 1994 (Public Law 103-417, DSHEA), authorized the establishment of the Office of Dietary Supplements (ODS) at the National Institute of Health (NIH). The ODS was created in 1995 within the Office of Disease Prevention (ODP), Office of the Director (OD), NIH. See Nutrition for Professionals Textbook page 266 for a description of the purpose and responsibilities of the ODS.
9	Although dietary supplements are regulated by the FDA as foods, they are regulated differently from other foods and from drugs. Classification as a dietary supplement is typically determined by the information that the manufacturer provides on the product label or in accompanying literature. There are no provisions in the DSHEA for FDA to "approve" dietary supplements for safety or effectiveness before they reach the consumer. Once a dietary supplement is marketed, FDA has to prove that the product is not safe in order to restrict its use or remove it from the market.
10	Drug manufacturers may claim that their product will diagnose, cure, mitigate, treat, or prevent a disease. Such claims cannot be made for dietary supplements. The label of a dietary supplement or food product may contain one of three types of claims; health claims, nutrient claims and structure-function claims. Health claims describe a relationship between a food, food component, or dietary supplement ingredient, and reducing risk of a disease or health-related condition. Nutrient content claims describe the relative amount of a nutrient or dietary substance in a product. A structure/function claim is a statement describing how a product may affect the organs or systems of the body, and it cannot mention any specific disease. Structure/function claims do not require FDA approval but the manufacturer must provide FDA with the text of the claim within 30 days of putting the product on the market. Product labels containing such claims must also include a disclaimer that reads, "This statement has not been evaluated by the FDA. This product is not intended to diagnose, treat, cure, or prevent any disease.
11	Standardization is a process that manufacturers may use to ensure batch-to-batch consistency of their products. In some cases, standardization involves identifying specific chemicals that can be used to manufacture a consistent product. Dietary supplements are not required to be standardized in the United States. In fact, no legal or regulatory definition exists in the United States for standardization as it applies to dietary supplements. Because of this, the term "standardization" may mean many different things.
12	Four categories of supplements include: plant based supplements, vitamin and mineral supplements, ergogenic aids, and weight loss supplements. See the Nutrition for Professionals Textbook pages 270 through 272 for details concerning each.
13	Eight categories of ergogenic aids include: water, carbohydrates/proteins, amino acids, anabolic steroids, creatine, caffeine, energy drinks, and energy bars. See Nutrition for Professionals Textbook pages 273 through 279 for the pros and cons of each.
14	Six categories of weight loss supplements evaluated by NCAAM include: acai, bitter orange, ephedra, green tea, sibutramine, mind and body approaches. See Nutrition for Professionals Textbook pages 279 through 282 for the pros and cons of each.
15	Three independent verification organizations include ConsumerLab.com, NSF International, and U.S. Pharmacopeia. See Nutrition for Professionals Textbook pages 273 through 279 for a discussion of each verification program.
16	Points to consider before ingesting dietary supplements include: It is safe; if safe is it effective; is it required; and what are the side effects. See Nutrition for Professionals Textbook pages 285 through 287 for details concerning each point.
17	See Nutrition for Professionals Textbook pages 289 through 293 for details concerning each organization and their position stand on the use of dietary supplements.

Answers

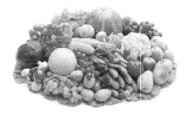

Incorporating Nutrition Programs

Performance Domain 2 - Answers
Incorporating Nutrition Programs

A. Prerequisites

Question	Answer
1	Dietitians have a degree in clinical nutrition and must obtain advanced education for recognition in specialty fields such as renal nutrition, pediatric nutrition, certified diabetes educator, certified nutrition support clinician, sports dietetics practice, gerontological nutrition practice and oncology nutrition practice. The basic educational requirement in a dietetics program is a bachelor's degree with a major in dietetics, foods and nutrition, food service systems management, or a related area. Students take courses in foods, nutrition, institution management, chemistry, biology, microbiology, and physiology. Other courses include business, mathematics, statistics, computer science, psychology, sociology, and economics. Individuals with the RD credential have fulfilled these requirements, possess at least a bachelor's degree (about half of RDs hold advanced degrees), have completed a supervised practice program, and have passed a registration examination, in addition to maintaining continuing education requirements for recertification.
2	A master's degree program in sports nutrition combines the fields of health and nutrition with fitness. Students learn ways to prevent injuries and provide treatment through nutrition programs. Master's degree graduates can obtain positions that focus on athletic performance and prevention of chronic diseases. A sports nutrition master's degree program teaches students how to measure metabolism, develop menus and create nutritional programs in order to prevent or accommodate injuries. Students also learn to customize specific training needs to improve physical performance in athletics. A masters degree in sports nutrition from a reputable university does not afford the same legal rights as a dietitian even though the individual with the masters degree in sports nutrition is clearly qualified to implement a sports nutrition program. Individuals who have earned a Masters Degree in sports nutrition from a reputable university cannot "sit in" for the Board Certified Specialists in Sports Dietetics (CSSD) exam (only RDs can take the exam); hence, they can not achieve the same legal status unless first obtaining a clinical dietetics degree.
3	State licensure regulations fall into the following categories: licensure, statutory certification, or registration. These terms are defined as: 1. Licensure statutes include an explicitly defined scope of practice and performance of the profession (nutrition/weight management) is illegal without first obtaining a license from the state. Hence, it is illegal to provide nutrition or weight management in these states without a license. There is a provision that allows a person to provide weight control services provided the program is developed and monitored by a licensed professional; and provided the individual does not change the program. 2. Statutory Certification limits use of particular titles to persons meeting predetermined requirements, while persons not certified can still practice the occupation or profession. Individuals in these states may provide weight management and nutrition services without being licensed; however, individuals may not use the term dietitian or licensed dietitian without adequate credentials. 3. Registration is the least restrictive form of regulation. Unregistered persons are permitted to practice the profession. Individuals in these states may provide weight management and nutrition services without being licensed.

4	Illinois is an example of a licensure law, CT is an example of certification, Texas is an example of the least restrictive form of regulation. See Nutrition for Professionals Textbook pages 339 to 341 for details concerning each type of licensure.
5	Choosing a qualified professional to oversee nutrition programs is of utmost importance. It must not be assumed that all dietitians have the appropriate background to provide this service. As discussed previously, a person may hold a master's degree in sports nutrition from a respected and reputable university but does not have the same legal rights as a licensed dietitian/nutritionist even though the individual with the masters degree in sports nutrition may be equally or more qualified to implement a sports nutrition program. Therefore it is important to interview potential licensed professionals to determine educational background, experience in nutrition program development, and experience in sports nutrition counseling.
6	The decision to pursue professional certification is an important step in being recognized as a competent practitioner in one's chosen discipline. The benefits of earning a certificate or certification in nutrition include: increasing level of expertise in the field of nutrition; adding a credential to list of credentials; providing additional services to help individuals become more successful; and increasing earning capacity. The first step when seeking a certificate or certification in nutrition is to decide on a regulatory program (such as an RD or CNS®). When seeking a nutrition certification from a non-regulatory program, research the program to confirm that it: adheres to all state licensure laws; includes all documents necessary to implement a nutrition program; possesses a defined scope of practice; offers continuous support by a qualified, licensed professional; and that the program provides mechanisms for the safety of the public.

B. Implementing Nutrition Programs

Question	Answer
1	See the Nutrition for Professionals Textbook pages 376 through 385 for details and the steps involve in the implementation of a nutrition program for individuals.
2	Body composition measures include Body Mass Index, waist-to-hip ratio, and percent body fat. See the Nutrition for Professionals Textbook pages 367 through 369 for more details.
3	The EER calculations for men 19 Years and Older: EER = [662 − (9.53 x Age)] + PA X [(15.91 x Weight) + (539.6 x Height)] Using the EER calculator at http://fnic.nal.usda.gov/fnic/interactiveDRI/, the EER for a 26 year old man who weighs 237 pounds, is 6 feet 4 inches tall and is "very active" is 4492 kcal/day. His body mass index is 28.9. This BMI is considered overweight which puts him at increased risk for disease. However, if this man is lean than the BMI would be an overestimate and he would not be at increased risk for disease.
4	Women 19 Years and Older: EER = [354 − (6.91 x Age)] + PA X [(9.36 x Weight) + (726 x Height)] Using the EER calculator at http://fnic.nal.usda.gov/fnic/interactiveDRI/, the EER for a 31 year old woman who weighs 132 pounds, is 5 feet 3 inches tall, and is active is 2328 kcal/day. Her BMI is 23.4 which puts her in the normal weight range and not at increased risk for disease.
5	It is important to structure a group program that includes a "curriculum" with learning objectives. A curriculum ensures that participants will complete the program with a new level of acquired information. Groups should be formed with common goals. An informational meeting is an excellent way to get the word out about your group program. Group meetings should contain similar topics as individual

	programs. See Nutrition for Professionals Textbook pages 386 and 387 for details on keys to a successful class.
6	Body Mass Index (BMI) is a number calculated from a child's weight and height and is a reliable indicator of body fatness for most children and teens. After BMI is calculated for children and teens, the BMI number is plotted on the CDC BMI-for-age growth charts (for either girls or boys) to obtain a percentile ranking. The BMI-for-age percentile is used to interpret the BMI number because BMI is both age-and gender-specific for children and teens. BMI-for-age weight status categories and the corresponding percentiles can be found in the Nutrition for Professionals Textbook on page 389 and 390.
7	See the Nutrition for Professionals Textbook pages 392 through 395 for details on how to establish a program for children and teens and includes the AASDN motivational placemats. Also see Stacy Teen client profile on page 411.
8	Nutrition programs for older individuals, athletes and vegetarians would be similar to programs for other adults except that each population has slightly different needs. The 50 to 70 year old must still face the battle of added weight gain and increased risk of chronic diseases associated with weight gain, while the over 70 year old faces decreased caloric intake associated with sarcopenia and are therefore at increased risk for nutritional deficiencies. Athletes require more calories, etc. See Chapter 5 in the Nutrition for Professionals Textbook for details on nutrient recommendations for athletes. Vegetarians may be low in some nutrients but most vegetarians can obtain most nutrients with a few possible exceptions such as iron and zinc. Strict vegetarians must obtain Vitamin B12 from fortified foods or supplementation since vitamin B12 is found only in animal products.

C. Promoting Success

Question	Answer
1	Dieting has been around for thousands of years and the history of dieting is a fascinating tale of how an entire industry can based on, and perpetuated on unscientific, misinformation. See the Nutrition for Professionals Textbook pages 422 through 426 for details.
2	The AASDN Beer and Prune diet is a "spoof" on diets in which Dr. Pentz uses steps outlined by Bonnie Liebman, of CSPI, to create a diet. Dr. Pentz puts the ridiculousness of diets into perspective. See the Nutrition for Professionals Textbook pages 427 and 428 for details; or visit www.bostonbeerprunediet.com.
3	As can be seen in the picture on page 429 in the Nutrition for Professionals Textbook, the beach ball and baseball weigh the same. But the beach ball and baseball are obviously very different in size. Hence, weight provides no information about size - only weight. Most Americans use the scale as a measure of determining size and health status. However, body composition is the appropriate measure to determine size. Also see page 429 for another example.
4	The Food and Drug Administration (FDA) is responsible for regulating most food products, while the United States Department of Agriculture (USDA) is responsible for regulating dairy, meat, and poultry products. Each organization developed labeling requirements that are unique to their respective products and requirements. The National Labeling and Education Act (NLEA) passed by Congress in 1990 required mandatory nutrition labeling to appear on most packaged foods regulated by the FDA. The NLEA pertains only to those labels of food products regulated by FDA, which has labeling authority over the majority of foods. However, meat and poultry product labels are under the authority of Food Safety and Inspection Service (FSIS) in the USDA, and alcoholic beverage product labels are

	under the authority of the Alcohol and Tobacco Tax and Trade Bureau of the Department of the Treasury, formerly the Bureau of Alcohol, Tobacco and Firearms. No regulations have been passed requiring the USDA to make meat and dairy labels comparable to the packaged food labels. This makes it very difficult for consumers to compare products. Prepackaged pizza with meat topping falls under USDA rules while cheese pizza is labeled according to FDA rules.
5	There are several factors in determining the content of whole grain in various products. • The definition "made with whole grain" does not specify an amount of whole grain the product must contain. Hence, the product can have "some" amount of whole grain or almost no whole grain. • "Made with whole grain" means a product may contain either a little or a lot of whole grain– a specified amount is not required. • "An excellent source of whole grain" means a product must contain at least 16 grams per serving or approximately nearly half of what most serving sizes are (30 to 55 grams). • "A good source of whole grain" means there can be as little as 8 grams per serving. Is this truly a good source when the product may be less than 50% whole grain? • "Multigrain" is a mixture of grains that can be mostly refined with minimal nutritional value. The definition of fat free includes the following: • If a serving size contains less than 5 calories, per serving it can be called "calorie free." • If a serving size contains 1/2 gram of fat, or less the product can be called "non-fat." • The nutrition label on a can of Pam fat free cooking spray reads: serving size 1/3 second, calories 0, calories from fat 0. A side panel compares the fat in the Pam spray to the fat in butter. In a one second spray, Pam has 7 calories while a tablespoon of butter has 104 calories. A low fat alternative to be sure, but 7 calories per second does not mean calorie free. The can contains 702 (1/3 second) servings, in other words, 234 seconds; hence, the can contains 1638 calories (234 seconds x 7calories/second). The labeling law states that if the serving size contains 1/2 gram of fat or less it can be called non fat, and if the serving size contains less than 5 calories per serving, it can be called calorie free. So the 1/3 second serving size fulfills the legal requirements. • Promise Ultra Fat-Free is 100% fat. • This same regulation holds true for "trans-fats." Many new products are not truly free of trans-fats. Organic is a labeling term that indicates: "the food or other agricultural product has been produced through approved methods that integrate cultural, biological, and mechanical practices that foster cycling of resources, promote ecological balance, and conserve biodiversity". Synthetic fertilizers, sewage sludge, irradiation, and genetic engineering may not be used. By definition, organic farming avoids the use of most artificial inputs, such as synthetic pesticides and fertilizers. Also banned are the use of animal byproducts, antibiotics, and sewage sludge, among other practices. The USDA has now defined the term gluten-free and foods containing this voluntary label must legally adhere to this definition. See pages 441 and 442 in the Nutrition for Professionals Textbook for the definition of gluten free.
6	Unlike nutrition information, health messages on labels were strictly forbidden until 1987. Since 1987, some scientifically based health statements have been permitted on labels subject to FDA approval. Health messages such as "Diets low in sodium may reduce the risk of high blood pressure," meant that the FDA had examined scientific evidence and reached the conclusion that there was a clear link between diet and health. Food manufacturers wanted to be allowed to inform consumers about possible benefits based on less than clear and convincing evidence. Food manufactures took their fight to court and the court ruled in their

		favor. The FDA must now allow claims that are **not** backed by convincing scientific evidence. There are now several "grades" of health claims that manufacturers can use. Unlike health claims, which require food manufacturers to collect scientific evidence and petition the FDA, structure-function claims can be made without any FDA approval. Manufacturers can add claims such as "improves bone health" or improves "cholesterol health" without any proof. However, manufacturers can not mention a disease or symptom. So claiming that a product "improves cholesterol levels" is illegal, but claiming that the product improves "cholesterol health" is legal. One can see how the public can be misled into believing product claims when no evidence exists.
	7	Examples of voluntary labeling include: free range, cage-free, natural, grass-fed, pasture-fed, pasture-raised, humane, no added hormones, and gluten-free. See the Nutrition for Professionals Textbook pages 441 through 442 for a discussion of each.
	8	The FDA does not evaluate or regulate terms placed on labels outside of the nutrition facts panel. The term "net carbs" does not have a legal definition and is not used by the FDA or the American Diabetes Association. The term "net carbs" came about when companies were seeking a way to market their products as being low in carbohydrates. Some food companies created the term "net carbs" and defined it as the total grams of carbohydrate minus the grams of sugar alcohols, fiber, and glycerin.
	9	Current agricultural policies are another contributing factor to the poor health of Americans. Government payments are skewed towards overproduction of commodity foods containing mostly processed, high calorie foods. Cheap commodities allow retailers and restaurants (and schools) to sell their products at a low cost. Not only are these commodities cheap, but farmers are also subsidized by the government which makes them lucrative crops to grow.
	10	See the Nutrition for Professionals Textbook pages 444 through 450 for sabotaging effects that hinder healthy lifestyles (eating out, portion distortion, too many calories in the evening, problem foods in the home, deprivation of favorite foods, shopping when hungry, eating by the numbers, friendly saboteurs, stress eating, traveling, meetings, holidays).

D. Building a Successful Nutrition Business

Question	Answer
1	The "EMyth," or Entrepreneurial Myth, is the flawed assumption that people who are an expert at a certain technical skill will therefore be successful running a business of the same kind.
2	See the Nutrition for Professionals Textbook pages 452 through 454 for factors to be considered before starting a business (money, passion, risk-taking, ethics, technology, tenacity, pros and cons).
3	Steps required in starting a business include: writing a business plan, identifying a location, completing the required state and federal regulations, deciding on a business type, obtain a federal EID number, establish a website, establish a separate bank account). See the Nutrition for Professionals Textbook pages 454 and 455 for more details.
4	Your business must reflect "you" and set you apart from others in your field. What is it that makes you unique? What is it that draws you to this profession? Success rests on your ability to differentiate your services from others. Your personal reasons are what will make your business different and successful. After answering these questions you are ready to go on to the next step.
5	Choosing your client base means deciding on which "type" of client you would like

	to work with. To answer this question, begin scripting an answer to what it is you do. It must be reiterated again if an individual is in the "precontemplative" stage, no changes will be made. This type of individual will "blame" you for their inability to live a healthier lifestyle. In working with a client that is not ready to change, he or she may likely attempt to blame you as the coach for their lack of success. You will simply be frustrating yourself and setting your business up for failure. There is no quicker way to destroy a business than this type of "bad" publicity.
6	Before deciding on pricing options, research other "diet" programs in your community. It's important to price your program relative to other programs in your area. One mistake many fitness professionals make is to price a nutrition program relative to personal training programs. The public pays much more for nutrition/diet programs than personal training. There is also hidden preparation time that must be included in your pricing scheme. A suggested pricing scheme is to multiply personal training rates in your area by 1.25 to 1.5. For example, if training rates average $50 an hour you should charge $62.50 to $75 per hour for nutrition services.
7	It's important to know what's available in your area that's competing for the same business. Some of the obvious services are Weight Watchers, fad diets, internet based programs, and the latest "best selling" book. Compare what you are offering to what's available. Look at all of the benefits of what you provide. Some examples might include individual attention, personal training, availability, experience, flexibility, and investment. It's important not to bad mouth your competition – the focus is what you offer that is unique to you – not what they don't offer. As part of your research, look into why some people are choosing other services. Are they offering something unique that you might want to add to your service or product line? Investigate the pricing structure. Typically clients are looking for the best "deal" not necessarily the lowest price. What makes your service a better deal to the client? Don't try to be all things to all people. Remember what you are offering, and stay true to your vision.
8	A limited budget just means you have to think a little more creatively. Consider launching your marketing campaign by doing one of the following: • Call your vendors or associates, and ask them to participate with you in co-op advertising. • Take some time to send your existing customers' referrals and buying incentives. • Have you thought about introducing yourself to the media? Free publicity has the potential to boost your business. By doing this, you position yourself as an expert in your field. • Invite people into your place of business by piggybacking onto an event. Is there a "race" coming to town? Are you willing to help? It could mean free publicity. • When you do spend money on marketing, do not forget to create a way to track those marketing efforts. You can do this by coding your ads, using multiple toll-free telephone numbers, and asking prospects where they heard about you. This enables you to notice when a marketing tactic stops working. You can then quickly replace it with a better choice or method. • By being diligent in your marketing and creating an easy strategy, such as holding yourself accountable to contact ten customers or potential customers daily five days a week, you will see your business grow at an exceptional rate. The great thing is it will not take a large marketing budget to make it happen.
9	See the Nutrition for Professionals Textbook pages 462 through 464 for components necessary to mount a successful advertising campaign.

Answers

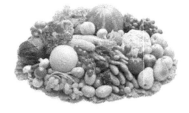

Communication /
Coaching Skills

Performance Domain 3 - Answers
Communication/Coaching Skills

A. Coaching Skills

Question	Answer
1	Coaching is a co-creative partnership between a qualified coach and a willing client that supports the client through desired life changes. The key to this definition is the term "co-creative." In coaching, you are not the expert in your client's life. You work with your client to discover solutions to their wellness challenges as they emerge through discussion and exploration.
2	A major difference between counseling and coaching is the client population. Coaches work with clients who are reasonably healthy and well-functioning and wish to augment their well-being through achieving certain personal or professional goals. Goals may be specific to wellness or performance or may be more broadly aimed at achieving greater life satisfaction through, for example, changes in career or lifestyle. The work is focused on the present and its influence on the future. The work is also typically brief and designed to accomplish the client's goals relatively quickly. "Improvement" and "enhancement" are hallmarks of coaching. Counselors also work with such clients and, when they do, there can be considerable overlap between coaching and counseling. However, counselors also work with clients who have some degree of impairment in functioning, ranging from mild to severe and this is when counseling enters areas not included in coaching. For example, along with various other aspects of their work with these clients, counselors may see a connection between the clients' present and past and may help clients explore early family relationships, previous traumatic experiences, or other aspects of the past in order to aid them in resolving present-day concerns. Counselors frequently help clients to deal with troubling thoughts and feelings, developmental concerns, and relationship issues. Such work may take considerable time, even extending to months or years. "Healing" and "recovery" are hallmarks of counseling.
3	Listening is an "art." It requires you to silence the expert in your brain, and focus on what's being said by the client. When listening, first, connect fully with the client. In order to do this, you must believe in your client's ability to effect change as he/she takes steps toward goal achievement. Next, you must be "present." You must not think, plan, or wonder while the client is speaking: your job is just to listen. It's surprising what you can hear people say when your history, knowledge, and assumptions are put aside. Finally, keep in mind that silence is valuable in many coaching moments. Give clients time to process questions and information, and arrive at their own conclusions. Remember, in successful coaching, the client has the answers. The coach is simply a partner that supports a willing client through desired lifestyle changes.
4	The Stages of Readiness to Change include the precontemplative stage, contemplative stage, preparation stage, action stage, maintenance stage, and relapse/recycling stage. See the Nutrition for Professionals Textbook pages 348 through 351 for details on each stage and its importance in the coaching process.
5	The change process refers to the the fears and difficulty associated with making lifestyle changes. See the Nutrition for Professionals Textbook pages 352 through 354 for a discussion concerning the process of change.
6	The SMART rules refers to an acronym associated with setting goals and objectives. S stands for specific—the goal must be specific. If the goal is too broad, it will

		be beyond achievement. <u>M</u> stands for measurable—the goal must be measurable. One can set goals, but if they are not measurable there is no way of knowing if that goal has been achieved. <u>A</u> stands for "A value"—the goal must be important and of value to the client. If not important, then it will not be accomplished. For example, a client losing weight for a spouse will not work. The client must set a goal that is important to him or her. <u>R</u> stands for realistic—the goal must be realistic. For a person who is 50% body fat, achieving 20% body fat in 6 months is unrealistic and will only frustrate the client. <u>T</u> stands for time frame—all goals must have a deadline. If no deadline exists, then there is no incentive to achieve the goal. The SMART rule helps clients set goals and objectives that are reasonable and not overwhelming.
	7	In coaching, support refers to an "unconditional positive regard for the client". A coach must show a genuine interest in a client's goal achievement. As the coach, you must be as highly invested in your client's success as he/she is. Show your client that you are invested by staying present when he/she speaks to you. Focus solely on what the client is saying and how he/she is feeling at any given moment; never lose yourself in your own thoughts or feelings. This requires practice. In the end and you will begin to feel what it is truly like to hear and care about what your clients are going through as they wade through the murky waters of change. Part of showing you care is holding your client accountable for his/her choices and actions. If he/she lets her weekly goals go unaccomplished or starts blaming and making excuses for missed opportunities to try new actions, don't let those moments slip by unnoticed! Coaching requires that you call your client on his/her dropped goals. Ask the client what he/she thought would happen by not following goal action steps, and ask what they experienced as a result. Holding clients accountable shows that you care. It communicates that you want them to have every opportunity to succeed, and you know that the client can't succeed if he/she doesn't try the new actions that he/she set out to try.

Answers

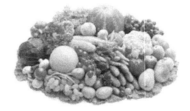

Nutrition Research / Application and Methods

Performance Domain 4 - Answers
Nutrition Research/Application Methods

A. Bias and Conflict of Interest

Question	Answer
1	When conducting research, scientists follow what is known as the "scientific method". This method relies on identifying and researching a problem to be solved or asking a specific question to be answered. The next step is to formulate a possible solution to the problem or an answer to the question (hypothesis) and make a prediction that can be tested through research. A study design is decided upon, the research is completed, and the data is collected. The data must then be analysed and the results interpreted. The original hypothesis is either supported by the data or is not supported. Scientists typically raise more questions so future research projects always exist.
2	The scientific method minimizes bias. Bias is defined as any tendency which prevents unprejudiced consideration of a question. In research, bias occurs when error is introduced into sampling or testing by selecting or encouraging one outcome or answer over others. Some degree of bias is nearly always present in a published study and can occur at any phase of the research project, including the study design, data collection, data analysis, and publication. Interpretation of bias cannot be limited to a simple yes or no. Instead, reviewers of the literature must consider the degree to which bias was prevented by proper study design, implementation, and conclusion. For clinical trials and randomized controlled trials, monitoring by a monitoring board (Data and Safety Monitoring Board) may be required. Vigilance is always necessary.
3	A conflict of interest involves the abuse of the trust that people have in research. A relationship based on trust is necessary with colleagues, the government, the study sponsors, and the public. A conflict of interest can damage an entire project which is why conflicts of interest are so serious.
4	Conflicts of interest are divided into two categories, intangible - those involving academic activities and scholarship; and tangible - those involving financial relationships. See the Nutrition for Professionals Textbook pages 309 through 312 for details concerning each category.
5	Before 1980, the federal government retained the rights to research and discoveries of the investigators it funded. At the same time, biotech companies were having difficulty obtaining licenses to manufacture and market their discoveries, and the research enterprise was not thriving. Congress responded in 1980 by passing the Bayh-Dole Act. The Bayh-Dole Act removed the ban on academic entrepreneurship and allowed researchers to take an active role in the private applications of their research. This enabled researchers and universities to benefit significantly from the shared royalties. Ultimately, many universities have thrived on these relationships; "...among companies that sponsor academic research, 58% require their investigators to withhold results for more than six months to give them time to apply for a patent or to provide a lead over competitors...". Potential or actual financial conflicts of interest are the unintended consequences of the Bayh-Dole Act.
6	Since 1980 with the passage of the Bayh-Dole Act, there has been a change within the research community where commercialization of biomedical research has become accelerated. Research and development by pharmaceutical companies increased 24 fold in 25 years (1977 to 2002), and these companies alone spent more on research and development than the total 2002 NIH operating budget of $24 billion. The number

		of physicians involved in drug studies increased by 60% during a five-year span. In the same time period, the proportion of trials conducted in academic medical centers dropped from 80% to 40%.
	7	In 1985, responding to the change created by the Bayh-Dole Act, the US Public Health Service, which includes the NIH and the National Science Foundation (NSF), enacted regulations entitled *Responsibility of Applicants for Promoting Objectivity in Research*. These regulations require institutions to establish standards and procedures that ensure that the design, conduct, or reporting of research is not biased by any conflicting financial interests of the investigator.
	8	It is clear that conflicts of interest are here to stay! Intangible and tangible conflicts of interest will always exist. In 2012, Fang and colleagues published a detailed review of the 2,047 retracted biomedical and life-science research articles indexed by PubMed. Of the articles retracted, 67.4% of the restrictions were because of misconduct, which includes fraud or suspected fraud (43.3%), duplicate publications (14.2%) and plagiarism (9.8%), miscellaneous reasons or unknown causes accounted for the reminder. Even after the articles are retracted, it is common for these articles to still be referenced in other articles. This highlights the importance of always tracking down the primary source. As the investigators of this study point out, "given that most scientific work is publicly funded and that retractions because of misconduct undermine science and its impact on society, the surge of retractions suggests a need to reevaluate incentives driving this phenomenon." The investigators also list possible solutions, which include: using checklists by authors and reviewers, improved training in logic, enhanced statistics, more focus on ethics, database for scientific misconduct, uniform guidelines for retractions, and a new reward system for science. Bekelman, et al. state that "most conflicts of interest created by academic-industry relationships are real, consequential, but tolerable, so long as they are managed to contain risks while preserving benefits. We must be vigilant against conflicts of interest that lead to bias and loss of objectivity. The enterprise of research depends on it.

B. Critical Analysis of Research

Question	Answer
1	The two major types of study designs are descriptive and analytical. See the Nutrition for Professionals Textbook pages 315 through 319 for a detailed description of study design including strengths and weaknesses of each.
2	Points for all professionals and consumers alike to consider when analyzing research can be found in the Nutrition for Professionals Textbook pages 320 to 323.
3	Reputable nutrition sources that can be trusted to provide minimally biased research and also addresses conflicts of interest include: 1. US Department of Agriculture Food and Nutrition Information Center. The USDA site http://fnic.nal.usda.gov has more than twenty-five hundred links to dietary, nutrition, diet and disease, weight and obesity, food-safety and food-labeling, packaging, dietary supplement, and consumer question sites. Using this interactive site, you can find tips and resources on how to eat a healthy diet and a food planner, among other sections. 2. The Academy of Nutrition and Dietetics (AND). The AND promotes scientific evidenced-based, research-supported food and nutrition information on its website, http://www.eatright.org. It is focused on informing the public about recent scientific discoveries and studies, weight-loss concerns, food safety topics, nutrition issues, and disease prevention. 3. Department of Health and Human Services. The HHS website, HealthFinder.gov, provides credible information about healthful lifestyles and the latest in health news. A variety of online tools assist with food-planning, weight maintenance, physical activity, and dietary goals. You can also find

healthful tips for all age groups, tips for preventing disease, and on daily health issues in general.

4. <u>Centers for Disease Control and Prevention.</u> The Centers for Disease Control and Prevention (http://www.cdc.gov) distributes an online newsletter called *CDC Vital Signs*. This newsletter is a valid and credible source for up-to-date public health information and data regarding food, nutrition, cholesterol, high blood pressure, obesity, teenage drinking, and tobacco usage.

5. <u>Dietitians of Canada.</u> Dietitians of Canada, http://www.dietitians.ca/, is the national professional association for dietitians. It provides trusted nutrition information to Canadians and health professionals.

6. <u>Health Canada</u>. Health Canada, http://www.hc-sc.gc.ca/index-eng.php, is the Federal department that helps Canadians improve their health. Its website also provides information about health-related legislation.

7. <u>Universities</u>. Several universities have excellent health letters that may be accessed on line. These health letters summarize the latest nutrition data. In most instances these universities, along with Center for Science in the Public Interest, agree on the latest nutrition research findings. It is this "consensus", along with multiple research studies indicated similar results which provides credence to the reported results. As evidence accumulates, scientists begin to integrate the findings which then become accepted among the nutrition community. Over the years, the picture of what is "true" gradually changes, and dietary recommendations are then reviewed and changed.

8. <u>Associations</u>. Associations such as the American Heart Association, the American Cancer Society, and the American Diabetes Society have helpful information for populations with these diseases. American College of Sport Medicine and National Strength and Conditioning Association have helpful information on sports nutrition.

9. <u>Medline/PubMed Resources Guide</u>: An excellent place to start a search for peer-reviewed literature.

10. <u>Google Scholar</u>: Provides for a literature search across many disciplines and includes theses, books, abstracts, and articles.

Answers

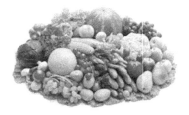

Professional and Legal Practices

Performance Domain 5 - Answers
Professional and Legal Practices

A. AASDN Professional Code of Conduct

Question	Answer
1	AASDN requires recertification of the Nutrition Specialist certification every two years. All Nutrition Specialists are required to obtain 15 contact hours every two years. All AASDN Certificants are held to higher standards since all Certificants are members of the health community. Therefore, AASDN-BOC has instituted a random audit whereby 10% of all Nutrition Specialists will be asked to provide documentation of contact hours. No fees are associated with this process. Certificants that are chosen are notified via USPS and must show proof of contact hours within 60 days of notification.
2	All Nutrition Specialists are required to renew their Nutrition Specialist Certification annually which includes a fee. Nutrition Specialists have the option to switch between 2 membership options: • Basic Membership. Benefits include entry into the NS member center which includes all documents needed to incorporate a nutrition program. Documents include: administrative documents, caloric needs assessment sheet; legal waiver, physician release form, responsibility agreement; ten session outline; individual scripted program, group scripted program, youth program, athletes and vegetarian program; menu plans, goal setting sheet and more. • Benefits also include AASDN product discounts and listing on the AASDN NS state page. • Benefits also include unlimited access to a sports dietitian. • The Basic Membership annual fee is $35. • Nutrition Manager Membership. All Nutrition Specialists have the option to upgrade to the Nutrition Manager Membership at any time. This option includes all the benefits of the basic membership and also includes the ability to provide more specialized services. AASDN professionals not only answers all questions, but also provide monitoring of client programs. For more details on this membership see Nutrition Manager at www.aasdn.org. The membership fee for Nutrition Manager is $299 annually.
3	AASDN requires a total of 15 contact hours every two years. Content must fall within the domains listed on page 17 in this study guide. AASDN also accepts documentation of work in the field of nutrition such as nutrition classes, lectures, etc. Certificants must complete the Continuing Education Course Petition form for approval of work completed in the field of nutrition. Nutrition Specialists are not required to recertify until the following reporting period. For example, a certificant that successfully completed the Nutrition Specialist exam in 2014 is not required to recertify until the 2017 reporting period. See pages 17 and 18 in this study guide for more details.

B. AASDN Scope of Practice

Question	Answer
1	"Wellness professionals" refers to individuals that practice health in the context of a healthy balance of the mind, body, and spirit that results in an overall feeling of well-

	being and excludes licensed dietitians/nutritionists. "Fitness professional" refers to both health related and skilled related fitness professionals. "Athletic Trainers'" refers to individuals that meet the requirements of a state licensing board and qualifications set by the Board of Certification. Athletic Trainers' are under the direction of a physician and are recognized by the American Medical Association; and are in good standing with the Board of Certification and their state licensing board. "Nutrition Specialist" refers to a person who has successfully completed the AASDN Nutrition Specialist program and is a member in good standing with the AASDN Credentialing Commission.
2	A "medical condition" is a broad term that includes all diseases and disorders.
3	See pages 21 and 22 in this study guide for a list of 10 points associated with the AASDN Code of Ethics.
4	The practice of nutrition education in conjunction with fitness/wellness programming by AASDN Nutrition Specialists includes a variety of educational activities/documents but only when created by, reviewed by, and/or in consultation with an AASDN licensed dietitian/nutritionist. No program/document change can be initiated without prior approval by an AASDN licensed dietitian/nutritionist. No program/document can be modified or altered in any way without approval by an AASDN licensed dietitian/nutritionist. The AASDN Nutrition Specialist, in conjunction with the AASDN licensed professional, may provide clients with educational information through lectures, articles, and classes. The AASDN Nutrition Specialist, in conjunction with the AASDN licensed professional, may utilize AASDN approved documents with the apparently healthy, exercising population. Nothing in this standard authorizes the AASDN Nutrition Specialist to "diagnose" disease or make nutritional recommendations for individuals requiring special dietary needs. Nothing in this standard authorizes the AASDN Nutrition Specialist to provide such services without direct approval and in consultation with an AASDN licensed dietitian/nutritionist. The AASDN Nutrition Specialist **cannot** provide nutrition services to individuals with medical conditions without direct oversight and in consultation with an AASDN licensed dietitian/nutritionist through the Nutrition Manager program.
5	An AASDN Nutrition Specialist cannot make any changes to any of the AASDN documents. No program/document change can be initiated without prior approval by an AASDN licensed dietitian/nutritionist. No program/document can be modified or altered in any way without approval by an AASDN licensed dietitian/nutritionist (standard 3).
6	AASDN requires recertification of the Nutrition Specialist certification every two years. All Nutrition Specialists are required to obtain 15 contact hours every two years. All AASDN Certificants are held to higher standards since all Certificants are members of the health community. Therefore, AASDN-BOC has instituted a random audit whereby 10% of all Nutrition Specialists will be asked to provide documentation of contact hours. No fees are associated with this process. Certificants that are chosen will be notified via USPS and must show proof of contact hours within 60 days of notification.
7	AASDN does not endorse any particular supplements or brand of supplements. It is beyond the scope of practice for Nutrition Specialists to recommend or suggest the use of any nutrition supplementation (vitamin, mineral, herbal, ergogenic, or weight loss). Any such recommendations must come directly from the client's physician or a licensed dietitian.
8	The Nutrition Specialist must refrain from endorsement of, or sales of, supplements and products containing supplement on the label. Such endorsement or sales constitutes a conflict of interest and is beyond the scope of practice of a non-licensed professional.
9	The AASDN Nutrition Specialist shall practice only within the boundaries of their competence as defined by their academic training, hands-on experience, professional certification, and in conjunction with a licensed dietitian/nutritionist. When indicated,

		the AASDN Nutrition Specialist professional shall monitor his/her effectiveness and take steps including, but not limited to, continuing education to maintain a reasonable level of awareness of current scientific and professional information. The AASDN Nutrition Specialist that has attained the AASDN Nutrition Specialist Certification who is in good legal and professional standing with all academic and certificate programs may implement programs that have been created by an AASDN licensed dietitian/nutritionist when working with the apparently, healthy exercising population. It is the responsibility of the AASDN Nutrition Specialist to be aware of specific statues in his/her state as well as understanding his/her professional standard of care and limitations in working with at risk populations or individuals with medical conditions.
10		Each certified Nutrition Specialist must provide professional service and demonstrate safe and effective client care in their practice. Each member shall: • Abide by the AAASD-BOC Professional Code of Conduct, including but not limited to, refraining from illegal use of terms such as dietitian and nutritionist. • Abide by the AASDN-BOC Scope of Practice. Including, but not limited to, using materials developed by qualified professionals and refraining from recommending or selling supplements which is beyond the scope of practice for all Nutrition Specialists. • Treat each colleague and/or client with the utmost and dignity and dignity and not make false or derogatory assumptions concerning their practice. • Refer clients to the appropriate medical practitioner when the Nutrition Specialist becomes aware of any change in the client's health status or medication; become aware of an undiagnosed illness, injury, or risk factor; become aware of any unusual client eating behaviors. Also refer the client to appropriate health care provider when supplemental advice is requested. • Remain in good standing and maintain current certification status by acquiring all necessary continuing education requirements.
11		Each certified Nutrition Specialist shall respect the confidentiality of all client information. In his/her professional role, the Nutrition Specialist shall: protect the client's confidentiality in conversations, advertisement and any other arena unless otherwise agreed upon by the client in writing or due medical and/or legal necessity; protect the interests of clients who are minors by law or unable to give voluntary consent by securing the legal permission of the appropriate third party or legal guardian; store and dispose of client records in a secure manner.
12		Each Nutrition Specialist must practice with honesty, integrity and lawfulness. The Nutrition Specialist shall: Maintain adequate and truthful progress notes for each client; accurately and truthfully inform the public of services rendered; honestly and truthfully represent all professional qualifications and affiliations; advertise in a manner that is honest, dignified and representative of services that can be delivered without the use of provocative and/or sexual language and or pictures.
13		AASDN-BOC may revoke or otherwise take action with regard to the application or certification of an individual in the case of: a) Ineligibility for certification b) Irregularity in connection with any certification application or examination. c) Unauthorized possession, use, access or distribution of certification examinations, score reports, answer sheets, certificates, Certificant or applicant files, documents or other materials. Material misrepresentation or fraud in any statement to AASDN or in any statement to the public in connection with professional practice, including, but not limited to, statements made to assist the applicant, Certificant, or another to apply for, obtain or retain certification. d) Negligence or malpractice in professional work, which includes, but is not limited to, the release of confidential medical information of clients or others with whom the Certificant or applicant has a professional relationship. e) The conviction of, plea of guilty or plea of no contest to a felony or

		misdemeanor, which is directly related to public health, athletic care or education. This includes but is not limited to rape, sexual abuse of a child, adult, or athlete, actual or threatened use of a weapon of violence; the prohibited sale or distribution of controlled substance, or its possession with the intent to distribute.
	f)	Not adhering to the eligibility requirements for certification candidacy, including breach of exam security; or not adhering to the continuing education requirements.
	g)	Not adhering to the Professional Code of Conduct and Scope of Practice.
	h)	Not cooperating with AASDN and/or AASDN Credentialing Commission investigations into alleged illegal or unethical activities. This would include but is not limited to, not cooperating with appropriate committees by withholding information, not responding to requests for information in a timely manner, or providing misleading information to an AASDN committee or individual member.
	i)	Engaging in conduct that includes, but is not limited to, unauthorized use of the AASDN name to endorse any products or services without proper authority or exploitation of a client for financial gain.
14	See pages 27 and 28 in this guidebook for details concerning the AASDN complaint, appeals, and sanctions process.	

Part 4
Study Activities

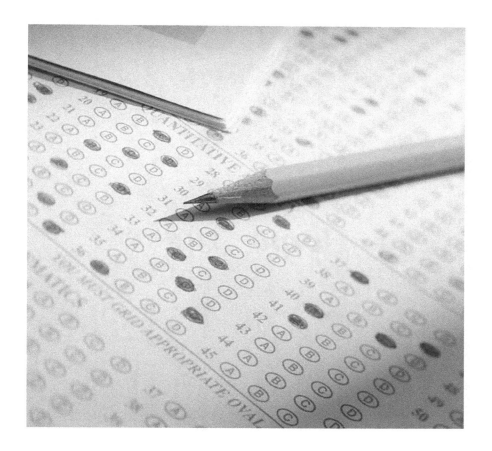

AASDN NS Certification

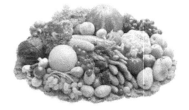

Home Study

AASDN Nutrition Specialist Home Study Option

The Nutrition Specialist Home Study option includes: The Nutrition for Professionals Textbook which serves as the official textbook for the Nutrition Specialist Certification; the AASDN Nutrition Specialist Certification Study Guide; a free online practice exam; 24 AASDN contact hours; and the Nutrition Specialist Exam.

This section contains information for students that have purchased the AASDN Nutrition Specialist Home Study option. Students that have purchased this option will receive additional support through input from AASDN staff on each assignment.

All other students are welcome to take advantage of these assignments; however, assignments will not be corrected, or commented upon, and no CEC's will be issued.

Directions for students that have purchased the Home Study Option!

1. Complete the assignments for each of the 5 domains.

2. Submit the assignments for each domain separately and in order. Do not submit assignments for Domain 2 until you receive confirmation and comments on assignments for Domain 1.

3. Follow the same procedure for each assignment.

4. Before submitting assignments be sure that each assignment contains:
   - Your name, email address and the assignment domain
   - Assignments must be sent as PDF files

5. Submit each assignment to info@aasdn.org.

Domain 1 Assignments

1. Choose one of the following presentations:
   - Create a presentation (approximately 10 slides) on the energy nutrients including why carbohydrates are important, and amounts required; roles, types and amounts of lipids that are required; roles of proteins and amino acids, recommended protein intake and why excessive amounts of proteins are not advantageous.
   - Create a presentation on energy production and utilization (approximately 10 slides). Include the steps involved in energy production; factors involved in energy utilization; and the importance of nutrient timing.
   - Create a presentation (10 slides) on complimentary and alternative medicine. Be sure to include NCCAM, NCCAM classifications, ODS, regulations, standardization, supplement categories, points to consider before ingesting a supplement, and position stands by national organizations on supplement use.

2. Choose one of the following handouts:
   - Create a handout on determining the estimated energy requirements (EER) for both males and females and include the body fat adjustment calculation.
   - Create handouts on two of the diseases discussed in Chapter 6 – Nutrition and Disease.

3. Choose two of the following and create a table for each:
   - Create a table for water and include the following: metabolic roles, recommended intake, deficiency and toxicity symptoms.
   - Create a table for the water soluble vitamins and include the following for each vitamin: metabolic roles, DRI, tolerable upper levels, food sources, deficiency symptoms, and toxicity symptoms.
   - Create a table for the fat soluble vitamins and include the following for each vitamin: metabolic roles, DRI, tolerable upper levels, food sources, deficiency symptoms, and toxicity symptoms.
   - Create a table for the major minerals and include the following for each mineral: metabolic roles, DRI, tolerable upper levels, food sources, deficiency symptoms, and toxicity symptoms.
   - Create a table for the trace minerals and include the following for each mineral: metabolic roles, DRI, tolerable upper levels, food sources, deficiency symptoms, and toxicity symptoms.

Domain 2 Assignments

1. Choose one of the following presentations:
   - Create a presentation (approximately 10 slides) on the history of dieting and why diets don't work! You may want to create your own diet as well.
   - Create a presentation on labeling regulations (approximately 10 slides). Be sure to include: the differences between the USDA and the FDA regulations; the definitions of whole grain, fat free, organic, gluten-free; health claims; voluntary and unregulated labeling terms; and net carbs.

2. Choose one of the following:
   - Construct a handout of fad diets from the 1800's until the present day.
   - Create a handout on how you would explain why the scale does not indicate size.
   - Create a brochure and advertising postcard containing the elements described in Chapter 12.

3. Complete the following activity:
   - Analyze two programs that combine nutrition and exercise. What do these businesses have in common and what makes them different? Itemize how your program will be unique and different from these businesses.

4. Complete any two of the four case studies. Answer all of the following questions for each of the two case studies that you choose:
   - For each of the following case studies, read the Client Profile which includes background information; personal, medical, exercise information; disease and dietary history; and a one day food recall. For each case study provide the following information:
     i.   Identify the "Stage of Readiness to Change". Is this client someone you can help? Explain your answer.
     ii. Do the stated goals and objectives follow the SMART. Rule? Explain your answer.
     iii. Read the client profile and identify any "red flags" that might indicate a reason for collaborating with a licensed professional. Explain your answer.
     iv. Identify body composition results and activity level. Why was this activity level chosen?
     v.   Determine the estimated energy requirements (EER), and calculate the body fat adjusted EER (if applicable). An online calculator can be found at http://fnic.nal.usda.gov/fnic/interactiveDRI/.

vi.   How did you determine the recommended daily caloric intake?

vii.   How was the body fat adjusted daily caloric intake determined?

viii.   Read the one day food recall. Approximately how many calories is the person ingesting?

ix.   Discuss the caloric differences between the one day food recall and the EER. Does this individual have to increase or decrease calories? How much of a caloric change would you recommend?

x.   Identify key coaching opportunities keeping in mind lifestyle changes.

xi.   Using your expertise and coaching skills explain how you would present the results and assist the person in setting goals and objectives.

Case Studies

Case Study 1 – Sally Stressed

Name	Sally Stressed		Date	07/05/13

Background

Sally is a 28 year old single nurse who has always been overweight. During high school and college she was "big" but she gained more weight after a relationship of several years ended. She has been working with a trainer for 6months and has managed to lose 20 pounds but she has plateaued at 200 pounds. She is 5'10" tall. She strength trains 3 times a week with her trainer and does a cardio workout three times a week for 30 minutes. Sally has decided to seek your help with a nutrition program.

Signed Agreements

Legal Agreement	Yes	Responsibility Agreement	Yes	Par-Q or equivalent	Yes

Demographic Information

Street Address	555 Glenn Drive
City/Town	West Palm Beach
State/Zip Code	FL 33419
Telephone	555.555.5555
Emergency Contact	
Emergency Phone	

Personal History

Age	28	Blood Type	A positive	Smoker	No
Date of Birth	01/15/85	Wt at Heaviest	228	Ever Smoked	No
Gender	Female	Wt at Lightest	180	Date Quit	NA
Height	5'10"	BMI	28.7	Occupation	Nurse
Weight	200 lbs	Waist/Hip	0.95	Stress Level	6
		% Body Fat	43.00%	Activity Level	Low-Active

Physical Activity

Describe Exercise Program	Weight training 3x/week, cardio 3x/week for 30 minutes
For How Long	Working with trainer for 6 months

Limitations to Exercise	None
Comments	

Medical History

Seeing a physician for any reason?	No
Taking any medications? If so list under comments.	No
Taking any over-the-counter medications? If so list under comments.	No
Taking any supplements? If so list under comments.	No
Comments:	

Disease History*

Does the client have any health related issues?	No
Does the client have any known diseases?	No
Disease Risk:	
Is the client a male over the age of 45 or female over the age of 55?	No
Has a parent or sibling experienced a heart attack before the age of 65?	No
Does the client have high blood pressure, diabetes, high cholesterol?	No
Does the client have any known allergies? If so describe under comments.	No
Does the client have any known eating disorders	No
Comments	
* If the client has any medical issues, diseases, indicators of disease risk or allergies you must receive written permission from a licensed professional before working with this client.	

Dietary History

What is the client's largest meal?	Dinner
Does the client snack during the day?	Yes
If yes, what types of snacks?	Fruit, Candy, Cookies
Does the client eat after dinner?	Yes
If so, what types of snacks?	Fruit, Candy, Cookies
What size does the client consider his/her meals to be?	Medium

Does the client eat when stressed?	Yes
Does the client eat when depressed?	Yes
Does the client feel he/she has or ever had an eating disorder?	No
Comments	

One Day Food Recall

	Breakfast	Snack	Lunch	Snack	Dinner	Snack
Day 1	Coffee with cream, 1 cup Cheerios, 1 cup non-fat milk water	Medium banana, 16 almonds, water	Protein drink	Raisins, water	Baked potato, broccoli (1 cup), salad with ½ cup dressing, 3 oz turkey. glass of wine (6 oz)	Cheese and crackers, Diet Soda
Calories						
					Total Calories	

Stage of Readiness to Change/ SMART Goals

Stage of Readiness to Change	
Goals:	
S	
M	
A	
R	
T	
Comments	

Case Study 2 – Stacy Teen

Name	Stacy Teen		Date	07/20/13

Background

Two parents come to you for help with their daughter – Stacy who is 16 years old. She is a great high school basketball player, and they have dreams of her getting a basketball scholarship. The daughter is obese, and the parents want you to help her lose weight. However, after speaking privately with the Stacy, you find out that she hates basketball, and she doesn't think she's fat! Upon further investigation, you discover that she does not want to disappoint her father so she agrees to work with you.

Signed Agreements

Legal Agreement	Yes	Responsibility Agreement	Yes	Par-Q or equivalent	Yes

Demographic Information

Street Address	222 Teen Drive
City/Town	Boston
State/Zip Code	MA, 02132
Telephone	555.555.5555
Emergency Contact	
Emergency Phone	

Personal History

Age	16	Blood Type	B positive	Smoker	No
Date of Birth	01/20/97	Wt at Heaviest	260	Ever Smoked	No
Gender	Female	Wt at Lightest	150	Date Quit	NA
Height	6'2"	BMI	33.4	Occupation	Student
Weight	260 lbs	Waist/Hip	0.95	Stress Level	7
		% Body Fat	39.00%	Activity Level	Active

Physical Activity

Describe Exercise Program	No weight training, basketball almost every day
For How Long	Two years
Limitations to Exercise	None
Comments	Stacy says she doesn't like basketball, and her coach is always screaming at her. While talking to you she begins to cry.

Medical History

Seeing a physician for any reason?	No
Taking any medications? If so list under comments.	No
Taking any over-the-counter medications? If so list under comments.	No
Taking any supplements? If so list under comments.	No
Comments:	

Disease History*

Does the client have any health related issues?	No
Does the client have any known diseases?	No
Disease Risk:	
Is the client a male over the age of 45 or female over the age of 55?	No
Has a parent or sibling experienced a heart attack before the age of 65?	No
Does the client have high blood pressure, diabetes, high cholesterol?	No
Does the client have any known allergies? If so describe under comments.	No
Does the client have any known eating disorders	No
Comments	
* If the client has any medical issues, diseases, indicators of disease risk or allergies you must receive written permission from a licensed professional before working with this client.	

Dietary History

What is the client largest meal?	Dinner
Does the client snack during the day?	Yes
If yes, what types of snacks?	Fruit, Candy, Cookies
Does the client eat after dinner?	Yes
If so, what types of snacks?	Fruit, Candy, Cookies
What size does the client consider his/her meals to be?	Medium
Does the client eat when stressed?	Yes
Does the client eat when depressed?	Yes
Does the client feel he/she has or ever had an eating disorder?	No
Comments	

One Day Food Recall

	Breakfast	Snack	Lunch	Snack	Dinner	Snack
Day 1	No breakfast	ice cream sandwich	2 slices of pizza, 24 oz coke,	Snickers candy bar orange slices at practice water	Macaroni and cheese, 2 cokes	2 Snickers bars (Mon and Dad don't know)
Calories						
					Total Calories	

Stage of Readiness to Change/ SMART Goals

Stage of Readiness to Change	
Goals:	
S	
M	
A	
R	
T	
Comments	

Case Study 3 – Randy Runner

Name	Randy Runner	Date	08/01/13

Background

Randy is a 20 year old collegiate cross country athlete. Randy is going into his third year on the team and is getting pressure to improve on his times. As a result, his coach strongly advised him to meet with you to improve his eating habits. While somewhat reluctant, he recognizes he could make better choices when it comes to nutrition and mentioned he wants to learn more about what to eat after practice. The team is currently doing two-a-day practices with a 5:45 am and 3:30 pm practice. Randy rarely eats breakfast, usually consumes a large lunch, and eats snack food throughout the evening.

Signed Agreements

Legal Agreement	Yes	Responsibility Agreement	Yes	Par-Q or equivalent	Yes

Demographic Information

Street Address	13 Elm Street
City/Town	Kalamazoo
State/Zip Code	MI 49006
Telephone	555.555.5555
Emergency Contact	
Emergency Phone	

Personal History

Age	20	Blood Type		Smoker	No
Date of Birth	07/24/93	Wt at Heaviest	152	Ever Smoked	No
Gender	Male	Wt at Lightest	138	Date Quit	NA
Height	5' 8"	BMI	22	Occupation	Student
Weight	145 lbs	Waist/Hip	0.93	Stress Level	6
		% Body Fat	8.20%	Activity Level	High

Physical Activity

Describe Exercise Program	Two-a-day practices includes running and light weight training.
For How Long	3+ years
Limitations to Exercise	None
Comments	

Medical History

Seeing a physician for any reason?	No
Taking any medications? If so list under comments.	No
Taking any over-the-counter medications? If so list under comments.	No
Taking any supplements? If so list under comments.	No
Comments:	

*Disease History**

Does the client have any health related issues?	No
Does the client have any known diseases?	No
Disease Risk:	
Is the client a male over the age of 45 or female over the age of 55?	No
Has a parent or sibling experienced a heart attack before the age of 65?	No
Does the client have high blood pressure, diabetes, high cholesterol?	No
Does the client have any known allergies? If so describe under comments.	No
Does the client have any known eating disorders	No
Comments	
* If the client has any medical issues, diseases, indicators of disease risk or allergies you must receive written permission from a licensed professional before working with this client.	

Dietary History

What is the client's largest meal?	Lunch
Does the client snack during the day?	Yes
If yes, what types of snacks?	Chips, energy bars, sports drinks
Does the client eat after dinner?	Yes
If so, what types of snacks?	Chips
What size does the client consider his/her meals to be?	Medium
Does the client eat when stressed?	No
Does the client eat when depressed?	No
Does the client feel he/she has or ever had an eating disorder?	No
Comments	

One Day Food Recall

	Breakfast	Snack	Lunch	Snack	Dinner	Snack
Day 1	Skip	Energy bar	Pasta, red sauce, juice, garlic bread, cookie	16.9 oz. Gatorade,	Two slices of pizza, six buffalo wings	Chips
Calories		250	Large serving	110		200
					Total Calories	

Stage of Readiness to Change/ SMART Goals

Stage of Readiness to Change	
Goals	
S	
M	
A	
R	
T	
Comments	

Case Study 4 – Derrick Dunn

Name	Derrick Dunn		Date	08/25/13

Background

Derrick is a 53 year old CIO and internet consultant. He has a home gym and is extremely regimented about his eating and about his workout program. He lifts weights 5 days a week and runs a few miles 2 to 3 times a week, sprinting the last several yards back to his home. He filters his water; avoids certain food such as bottom feeding fish for their lack of dietary cleanliness; avoids sugars, HFCS, trans fats and food additives. He rarely eats out and he measures everything that he eats to exact quantities. He eats very small portions of food, despite the variety. Derrick is please with his lean look but would like to add muscle to his structure, without adding any fat. He is 5'9", weighs 143 pounds and his body fat is 10%. He likes a variety of fruit and vegetables (organic); prefers vegetarian protein sources, but will eat chicken and white fish, though it's not his favorite. He eats only organic grain and organic eggs.

Signed Agreements

Legal Agreement	Yes	Responsibility Agreement	Yes	Par-Q or equivalent	Yes

Demographic Information

Street Address	555 Dun Drive
City/Town	Chicago
State/Zip Code	IL, 60601
Telephone	555.555.5555
Emergency Contact	
Emergency Phone	

Personal History

Age	53	Blood Type	A positive	Smoker	No
Date of Birth	02/15/60	Wt at Heaviest	145	Ever Smoked	No
Gender	Male	Wt at Lightest	140	Date Quit	NA
Height	5'9"	BMI	21.2	Occupation	CIO
Weight	143 lbs	Waist/Hip	0.8	Stress Level	(h) 3 (W) 7
		% Body Fat	10.00%	Activity Level	Active

Physical Activity

Describe Exercise Program	Lifts weights 5 days a week and runs a few miles 2 to 3 times a week, sprinting the last several yards back to his home.
For How Long	Years
Limitations to Exercise	None
Comments	Derrick wants to get leaner but doesn't appear to eat very much.

Medical History

Seeing a physician for any reason?	No
Taking any medications? If so list under comments.	No
Taking any over-the-counter medications? If so list under comments.	No
Taking any supplements? If so list under comments.	No
Comments:	

Disease History∗

Does the client have any health related issues?	No
Does the client have any known diseases?	No
Disease Risk:	
Is the client a male over the age of 45 or female over the age of 55?	Yes
Has a parent or sibling experienced a heart attack before the age of 65?	No
Does the client have high blood pressure, diabetes, high cholesterol?	No
Does the client have any known allergies? If so describe under comments.	No
Does the client have any known eating disorders	No
Comments	
* If the client has any medical issues, diseases, indicators of disease risk or allergies you must receive written permission from a licensed professional before working with this client.	

Dietary History

What is the client largest meal?	Lunch
Does the client snack during the day?	Yes
If yes, what types of snacks?	Nuts and fruits
Does the client eat after dinner?	No

If so, what types of snacks?	
What size does the client consider his/her meals to be?	Small
Does the client eat when stressed?	No
Does the client eat when depressed?	No
Does the client feel he/she has or ever had an eating disorder?	No
Comments	

One Day Food Recall

	Breakfast	Snack	Lunch	Snack	Dinner	Snack
Day 1	Oatmeal, egg whites, coconut oil, banana, honey	Carrots, almonds, Banana	Vegetable soup, brown rice, Slim Fast, grapes,	Banana, glass of soy milk, organic organic orange juice, yogurt	Salmon, brown rice, corn, salad, olive oil PROLAB soy drink	
Calories						
					Total Calories	

Stage of Readiness to Change/ SMART Goals

Stage of Readiness to Change	
Goals:	
S	
M	
A	
R	
T	
Comments	

Domain 3 Assignments

Answer all of the following questions:

1. List 15 "how and what" questions that are effective in coaching.
2. List 15 questions that would not be effective coaching questions and explain why.
3. Describe a client who is ready to change and one who is not. What do they say? How do they act?
4. Initiate a conversation with a volunteer concerning a nutrition program that you are about to implement. Describe your program in detail. Using this opportunity use coaching skills, including listening and questioning, to determine this person's Stage of Readiness to Change. Summarize your conversation, indicate this person's Stage or Readiness to Change, and explain your answer.
5. Describe how you would work with a client who is in the relapse and recycling stage.
6. Identify a change in your own life that was challenging for you, and describe how you finally accomplished it. Cover the areas of goal-setting, practice, support, and your reasons for changing.
7. Give specific examples of how you would work with the following clients.
    i.   Lisa has just met her 3-month goals with you. She has been consistently working out at the gym 3 days a week for 45 minutes. She began doing yoga on Sunday and she loves it. She has started eating breakfast for the first time in her life. She is slowly weaning herself off of caffeine. She expressed a desire to begin learning how to buy and prepare healthy foods at home so she is not at the mercy of other people's high-fat, high-sugar foods. How would you work with Lisa on this new goal?
    ii. Mitch has been coaching with you for 5 months and he is still throwing the blame card around. He blames his wife for not helping him exercise, and he uses her as an excuse for his unhealthy eating habits—even at work. He has cut back significantly on his wine drinking since he started with you; he now takes the stairs at work instead of the elevator, but he seems to be stuck in this rut in regards to his unhealthy habits around his wife. He feels he has no support at home and therefore he is nearly ready to give up on his healthy goals. How would you coach Mitch out of his rut?
8. Would you work with the following clients in person or on the phone? Could you work with them in either manner? Why or why not?
    iii. Gloria is a 55-year-old obese woman who came to you to learn how to control her meal portions and start an exercise program. She is afraid of failing because she has tried every diet book in the bookstore and not one of them has worked for her. You discover that she has no idea how her

metabolism has been affected by years of dieting. She needs education and guidance as she explores options for finally getting healthy.

iv. Michael is a 35-year-old VP of a marketing company who works more than 80 hours a week. He puts his work and his company before everything else, and his health is paying the price. He has high cholesterol and high blood pressure, and he is on the verge of taking medication for both. His doctor told him he needs to start exercising and watching his diet, but Michael is reluctant to spend any time on himself at all.

9. Answer the following questions for the three clients below. Provide a one page summary on each.

- How would a personal trainer/athletic trainer work with this client, student, or patient? What might they focus on?
- How would a nutrition consultant?
- How would a therapist or counselor?

i. Maryanne is a single 55-year-old woman who is 75-pounds overweight, a smoker, and has a family history of diabetes. She is at high risk for the disease. Her doctor recommended she begin an exercise and nutrition program, and try to quit smoking. She has begun walking regularly but is having trouble sticking to it because she "gets bored." She says her entire family has been "heavy" as long as she can remember. She has only ever known the traditional meat and potatoes-type of dinner, and she says it's "impossible" to eat any other way. She drinks Coke at every meal, and she does not seem to understand that excess calories (not fat) are contributing to her weight gain.

ii. Tony is an 18-year old freshman in college who has recently lost a lot of weight through dieting. He does not want to gain the Freshman 15 or return to his prior obese self. He has been working out with his buddies, but they are all getting "cut" and he is still flabby. He comes to you to get leaner, but he has a deep fear of eating enough to sustain muscle growth. He is completely clueless about sports nutrition, even though he is a baseball player (pitcher) and he needs to sustain his energy for long games. He lives in the dorm and has to eat dorm food. Between running to classes and making all of his baseball practices and games, his eating habits are atrocious. His energy is generally low and he wants to improve that as well as his physique.

iii. Suzanne is 32-year-old married woman with a 3-year-old and a 14-month-old baby. She stays at home to take care of the kids. Her husband commutes to another city 4 days a week, and the two rarely see each other. She feels alone and overwhelmed with work around the house. Her eating habits have suffered since her husband is no longer around much and she only cooks "kid food," so she mainly relies on takeout—when she has time to sit down and eat. Her body fat has shot up from 18% before her first child to 32% after her second child, and she wants to reduce it by at least 10% for health and aesthetic reasons. She's having a hard time exercising because she feels totally alone in raising the kids, and none of her friends have kids yet so they don't really do much together anymore.

Domain 4 Assignments

Choose either one of the following two activities and answer all questions associated with the activity that you choose:

1. Choose an up-to-date nutrition research article published in a peer-reviewed journal and using the information provided on 320 to 322 critically analyze this article.

    i.   Determine bias and conflict of interest in this research article.

    ii. In a summary paper explain your answers to the questions listed on pages 320 to 322. Also explain your findings.

    iii. Conclude your paper by rating this article on a scale of 1 to 10. A score of 1 indicates poor quality and a score of 10 indicates excellent quality research with minimal bias and conflict of interest.

2. Choose a popular nutritional supplement and complete an online literature search of this supplement.

    i.   Using the information on page 323 in the Nutrition for Professionals Textbook indicate whether or not the websites describing this product are valid.

    ii. List the websites providing the information and list the references listed on the websites.

    iii. Using the same information to analyze a research article, investigate at least 2 of the references listed on these websites.

    iv. Determine bias and conflict of interest.

    v.   In a summary paper explain your answers to the questions listed on pages 320 to 322 for both of the 2 references you listed in iii. Also explain your findings.

    vi. Conclude your paper by rating your literature search on this supplement on a scale of 1 to 10. A score of 1 indicates advertising/non scientific research and a score of 10 indicates excellent quality research with minimal bias and conflict of interest.

Domain 5 Assignments

Answer all of the following questions:

1. Determine the licensure law in your state and explain how you will adhere to this licensure law.

2. A dietitian approaches you and indicates that it is illegal for you to provide nutrition services in your state. Create a response letter on why as an **AASDN** Nutrition Specialist you are legally qualified to provide nutrition services in your state (even if your state has strong licensure laws). You may also want to include information taken from the article written by Michael Ellsberg on pages 337 and 338 in the Nutrition for Professionals Textbook.

3. You have a potential nutrition client that has heart disease. Create a letter explaining to this client what options he/she has when working with you.

4. You witness another **AASDN** Nutrition Specialist altering online documents. What, if any, steps would you take?

5. You are approached by a national supplement company asking you to recommend and sell a new protein drink. This drink has been advertised in all the fitness magazines and clients in your gym are "raving" about their success in muscle hypertrophy due to this new drink. Create a letter responding to this company explaining your options as an **AASDN** Nutrition Specialist.

Part 5
NS Practice Exam
Questions

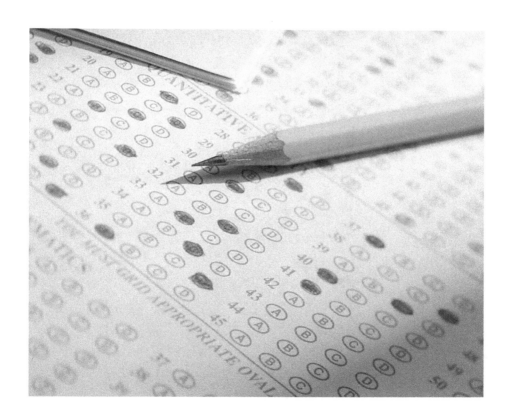

Practice Exam

Students may purchase an online practice exam. Students that have purchased the AASDN Nutrition Specialist Home study option may complete a practice exam free of charge. Visit http://www.aasdnstore.com/ and click on "Nutrition Specialist Exam". The next few pages contain examples taken from the online practice exam.

Question 1 of 100

A double-blind, placebo controlled, clinical trial is the "gold standard" in research design and results do not need to be viewed in the context of other published research.

- A) True
- B) False

Question 2 of 100

BMI may overestimate body fat in:

- A) Athletes and others who have a muscular build
- B) Anorexics and older individuals
- C) Athletes and anorexics
- D) Children and older adults

Question 3 of 100

After calculating the BMI in the previous example for the male who is 36 years old, 6 feet 7 inches tall, and weighs 235 pounds you determine that this man is considered obese according to the BMI norms.

- A) True
- B) False

Question 4 of 100

Homeostasis is

- A) Transamination of amino acids
- B) The maintenance of caloric needs
- C) The maintenance of constant internal conditions in body systems (balance)
- D) The maintenance of appetite

Question 5 of 100

Peristalsis is defined as:

- A) The layer of smooth muscle in the stomach
- B) The wavelike muscular contractions of the gastrointestinal tract that pushes its contents down the tract.
- C) The action of enzymes in the mouth
- D) The action of the pancreas in producing enzymes.

Question 6 of 100

Anabolism consists of reactions in which larger molecules are broken down into smaller molecules.

- A) True
- B) False

Question 7 of 100

Calories are defined as:

- A) The amount of water needed to produce heat
- B) The amount of heat necessary to raise the temperature of one kilogram of water by one degree centegrade
- C) The amount of heat necessary to produce boiling water
- D) The amount of energy required to heat one kilogram of water by one centegrade

Question 8 of 100

The role of dietary proteins is to provide the body with amino acids that the body can then use to synthesize required (internal) proteins. Proteins in the diet cannot affect protein synthesis (can only provide all the essential amino acids for protein synthesis)

- A) True
- B) False

Question 12 of 100

Absorption rate of carbohydrates depends on:

- **A)** Whether or not the carbohydrate is a simple sugar or polysaccharides; whether or not other nutrients such as fiber, fat and protein are present
- **B)** Whether or not the carbohydrate has a low glycemic response and a low glycemic load
- **C)** Whether or not the carbohydrate is raw or cooked
- **D)** Whether or not the carbohydrate is organic or gluten-free

Question 13 of 100

Insulin resistance is diagnosed by a blood test to determine insulin levels.

- **A)** True
- **B)** False

Question 14 of 100

The National Center for Complementary and Alternative Medicine (NCCAM) is:

- **A)** A regulating committee of the FDA
- **B)** Is a regulating committee assigned to oversee supplement manufacturing
- **C)** Is the federal government's lead agency for scientific research on complementary and alternative medicine
- **D)** Is a federal agency overseeing conflicts of interest

Question 15 of 100

A major reason for the "explosion" in sales of dietary supplements is due to the passage of the Dietary Supplement Health and Education Act of 1994.

- **A)** True
- **B)** False